MW01169716

STEEL

A Memoir

By

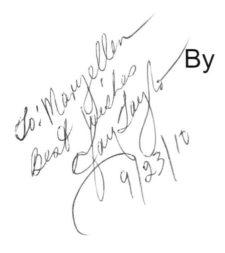

To: Maryellen
Best Wishes
Fay Taylor
9/23/10

Fay Taylor

Written by Fay Taylor 2008

Copyright© Fay Taylor

ISBN-10: 0-9800468-0-7
ISBN-13: 978-0-9800468-0-9

Library of Congress Control Number: 2008906700

Published by Taylor Productions
United States

Email: noproblem11@comcast.net

Printed in the U.S.A by
Morris Publishing
3212 East Highway 30
Kearney, NE 68847

First published 2008

To my family and relatives who have stood by me from the beginning

ACKNOWLEDGEMENTS

Special thanks to my dear friend and teacher Barbara Gershenbaum, who taught me how to be a good writer. For your patience and for being there to answer my questions many years after the class had ended.

To my dear sweet sister AlvaJoy, without you this book would not have been possible. I cannot thank you enough for the many hours you have spent editing my work while ignoring your family and home. God bless you.

Thanks also to my brother Hugh for choosing such a great title and cover design.

To my sister Shirley, thanks for your input, it made a difference in my writing.

Sister Georgia, your expertise with the medical information is greatly appreciated.

Kay, my niece, you sent the clown to cheer me up when I was down and your opinions in the beginning of my writing career were an asset. Thanks.

Thank you to my niece Dawn for doing the copyediting.

Credit and appreciation goes to my niece Jacqualyn for painting the cover from my x-ray.

My official editor, Vangella 'Vjange Hazle' Buchanan, thanks for your patience and assistance in guiding me through the publishing process.

Foreword

"I think a hero is an ordinary individual who finds strength to persevere and endure in spite of overwhelming obstacles"-Christopher Reeve

There are more than 250,000 people in the United States with traumatic spinal cord injury and Mrs. Fay Taylor is one of them. They are the real heroes as they battle to overcome the impairments from their injury every day of their life. Mrs. Taylor's story is not only about her grit and determination while dealing with the effects of her spinal cord injury, but a story of a true American immigrant.

The narrative features her great anticipation and delight as she leaves the island of Jamaica for the United States in the early 70s. Her early days in Jamaica, her successes and tragedies in the U.S. are poignant and heartwarming on one hand, gut wrenching and sad on the other. The memories of her tragic fall and injury are vivid and terrifying, but her ultimate struggle to heal and rehabilitate portrays the courage and faith of Fay and her close and supportive family.

Fay Taylor's story is a message of courage, determination, and hope, and will be an inspiration to all.

Subramani Seetharama, M.D., FAAPM & R
Director of Spinal Cord Injury Program and Medical Director of Eastern Rehabilitation Network Hartford Hospital, Hartford, Connecticut.

CHAPTER OUTLINE

CHAPTER 1

INTRODUCTION

I always wondered what it felt like the moment you realize you are about to die. I was about to find that out one late July day in the Pocono hills where my husband Charley and I had decided to sneak a quick weekend for a much needed getaway. To say I had a premonition of how the day would end would be stretching the truth. I really had no inkling how close to dying I would get that afternoon as we made the four hour drive to what I thought was going to be our escape to paradise.

Prior to 1989, I had felt blessed. Not rich, but comfortable: a decent home, a good job, a reliable car, a loyal husband, Charles, and three beautiful children, Charles Jr., Sean, and Monique. I even considered it a blessing having children of both sexes. Then, on one of those cloudless days in the middle of the summer of 1989, the water main of my life broke; challenges came gushing forth like water flowing into the streets. Nothing could have prepared me for the drastic changes that were about to determine my future and that of my family.

It was time for shift rotation in Information Management System (IMS) where I worked as a computer operator at one of the largest insurance companies in Hartford, Connecticut. Finally, a long weekend off; the kids were at camp for two weeks, and my husband, Charley suggested we take a mini vacation. It had been too long since we had had some time alone. A romantic weekend was just what we needed since our work schedules did not allow us much time to even see each other and, with three active kids, we were starting to look like the legendary two ships passing in the night. When we read the brochures for the beautiful Caesars Pocono Resorts in Lakeville, Pennsylvania we felt that this was the perfect place to go.

Excitement kicked in when we saw the variety of activities in which we would be able to participate: table games, swimming, and horseback riding. Finally, I would be able to fulfill my childhood dream of horseback riding, a dream that was born when my mother, Urceline, would take me to our weekly triple bill shows (three shows for the price of one) at the Ritz Theatre in Kingston, Jamaica, my homeland. I had fallen in love with both the on screen cowboys and their horses, and longed to ride a horse.

The date planned was July 28, 1989, our eldest son's birthday. It was hard deciding whether to stay and have a party for Charles Jr. but, since he was at camp, we thought this would be one of our few chances to get away by ourselves. We were scheduled to check in at 3:00 p.m. After what seemed like a long wait we, headed down 91 south and were finally on the road to the Pocono resort. Our home was left in the care of my sister, LaVerne who would water my plants and pick up the mail.

WEEKEND IN THE POCONOS

The drive to the Poconos was without event as Charley and I chatted companionably about nothing in particular. The sun was shining brilliantly as I leaned back in my seat, eyeglasses plugged to my face to minimize the glare. The sky was cloudless. We pulled up at the resort at one in the afternoon, a little too early to get our keys to our room so we decided to explore the area. We did some shopping at a little country store where I bought some t-shirts for the children and key chains for my sisters.

Stopping at the Indian Museum, we splurged on souvenirs and learned some new and interesting facts about American-Indian heritage. I was shocked to learn that the Pilgrims of early America had given clothing and blankets that were contaminated with Smallpox to the Indians as gifts, causing hundreds to die because the Indians had no cure for this disease or any immunity to it.

We hurried back to the resort by check-in time, picked up the keys and went to our room. We barely got in through the door. Charley and I made wild passionate love on the floor. How long had it been since we had had the freedom to do that? We then relaxed, wrapped in each other's arms, the cool breeze coming through the open window blowing over us, as we lay still, wanting to remain there forever. But suitcases had to be unpacked; reservations had to be made.

For dinner, I dressed in black evening wear, my dress bejeweled with rhinestones that glistened seductively on the collar and on the buckle of the wide belt around my waist. My body was still youthful and petite after three children. I wore high heels and carried a matching handbag. Charley looked elegant in his black suit with white shirt and floral tie, and into the bar we strolled, arms locking like young lovers.

We had a drink, and after making reservations for that night's show and dance, we went to dinner. Seated by the window, I was captivated by the breathtaking view of the lake, the trees, the beautiful flowers, and oh!! those swans, how gracefully they moved across the water. Dinner was buffet style, affording a casual atmosphere in which to mingle. We met a number of friendly and humorous couples, some of whom had had the same idea as we had, to get away for the weekend.

After dinner we went for a walk by the gorgeous lake over which the evening moon was shining. This, indeed, was heaven on earth. In the game room the jukebox was playing. It seemed like a scene from some movie. We played table tennis for the first time together. (It was my first time playing but Charley is an expert). Charley asked me to make a selection from the jukebox. He liked the songs that I had chosen and we both enjoyed the music while hitting the balls to the rhythm of our favorite songs. I lost, of course, and we left for the night's show and our great seats in the front row.

The comedy routine was hilarious. We could not restrain ourselves from laughing between sipping our drinks. Charley was the object of some of this humor as the Master of Ceremonies teased him when he tried to sneak unnoticed to his seat from the bathroom. After the show we danced until 2:30 a.m. We danced so much we made ourselves hungry again. The ham sandwich we had at a little fast food place in the same building revitalized our bodies and we walked back to our room, where we totally exhausted ourselves making love again, but this time on clean sheets and soft pillows. This night would go down as one of the best nights of our lives.

The next day, Saturday July 29th, we woke early and made love in the quiet of the morning. We played in the whirlpool for a while like two teenagers stealing their first time together, and then took a long shower together. We looked forward to a good breakfast as we read the newspaper and waited for room service. The meal, however, was disappointing; we would dine in the dining room the next day, we decided.

It was still early so we watched "The Birds," Alfred Hitchcock's classic. Before it ended, Charley suggested we start the day's activities. The first thing on the agenda was horseback riding. At approximately 10:30 a.m. we strolled out to the stables, inhaling the fresh air, and admiring the beauty of our surroundings. We were the first couple to arrive at the stables, and were told by the attendant to wait for the other couples because the ride was organized in groups. About three other couples showed up. My husband paid at a little shed while I waited in the shade of a big tree by the gate.

I watched in anticipation as two attendants brought out the horses one at a time and helped the others with their mounts. First, they mounted two couples, then one man. His wife made some attempts to get up on a giant white stallion named Toby but had difficulties mounting him, so she turned away and decided not to go riding. I was then instructed to mount Toby. I exclaimed with anxiety: "Me! I don't want to go on that horse, he is too big." The attendant replied, "He is a good horse." After being reassured, I mounted without fear and asked Charley to take my picture. My first question to the attendant was, "What should I do if he gallops?" She replied, "He won't, these horses don't do that." Her partner then gave me the riding instructions, which were simple, and I relaxed. Charley was next, and declined when I offered to take his picture.

When everyone was mounted the guide started the ride, leading the way along the narrow trail. The wet and muddy grounds at the beginning gave way to dry paths as we rode on. The golden rays of the sun shone through the lush green trees, and there was a certain peace in the country setting as we slowly rode through the shadows of the leaves with the cool breeze caressing our bodies. I whispered a short prayer thanking God for a lovely day and the fulfillment of my childhood dream. I had a fleeting thought about how I would share my riding experience with friends and family when I returned home.

I was enjoying the ride to the maximum. I wished all my family and friends could see me now. Maybe I would never ride like those cowboys of my childhood movies, but

I was finally riding. I could feel the power of the animal beneath me. Suddenly my easygoing horse tripped, his forelegs bent, throwing me forward. I realized, with horror that my right foot was out of the stirrup. I yelled, "There is something wrong with my horse!"

Everyone stopped and the guide came to help me. Thoughts of dismounting were immediately dismissed by fear of the horse stepping on me, so I waited with the hope that the guide would help me off. Toby, however, had other ideas. While trying to regain his footing, he tossed me to the ground. I felt myself falling as if in slow motion, just like in the movies. I never imagined that was how it really seemed. I felt no fear; I would get up. There was instant pain and shock, the shock of the vigorous way in which Toby had gotten up, and the impact of my hitting what I later realized was a rock. I could not move.

Since I didn't lose consciousness, I was fully aware from the moment of impact that I could not move. My lower body felt crushed inside and out. There was a burning sensation in my bladder, along with severe tearing pain in my lower back, followed by numbness, which slowly crept along my thighs and legs to the tip of my toes. Within minutes there was no sensation in my legs. Was this the prelude to my death?

"O God!" I yelled, "I can't move! ... Charley help me!" He said he had to wait for the guide to help him off his horse. I had fallen on the trail, so the guide and Charley tried to move me to let the other riders pass. I screamed like a banshee as they tried to move me and they gave up. Charley then knelt next to me to protect me from the horses while the other riders passed, hoping he would not be stepped on.

For about an hour, I lay on the ground in the position in which I had fallen, unable to move and in excruciating pain, with Charley by my side taking pictures while the guide went for help. The wait was as painful as the sensations ripping through my body. My thoughts raced out of control. Paralysis? Death? My future? Surely death was staring right at me and I was staring back. Why was the ambulance taking so long to get here? I asked Charley what he thought. "I don't know, Fay" he replied. Being in extreme pain and discomfort, I placed my right hand underneath my back to ease the pain. It did not help, and I could not remove it due to the intensity of the pain, so there it stayed until the ambulance arrived.

Finally, I felt hands gently rolling and lifting me,

while I screamed in pain. The sound of the sirens told me I was on my way to the hospital. The realization that I was now the patient hit me and I was overcome by a strange feeling. I had never thought about the person inside an ambulance before, now that person was me.

ON BEING A PATIENT

At the Pocono Medical Center, my anticipation of getting relief from the excruciating pain was crushed like my back, when they told me that I could not have medication until the extent of the injuries was known. When finally the extent of the injury became known, I would not be able to be helped at this small local hospital. The helicopter must have been waiting because I was immediately taken onboard, and transported to the Thomas Jefferson University Hospital in Philadelphia. Charley said he rode in the front of the ambulance, but he had denied my request to accompany me on the helicopter. Later he told me he did not go on the copter because he knew he had no way of returning to the resort from the hospital. But he did remember to use the camera and take more pictures of me being pushed to the copter.

The three people on the copter were the pilot, a nurse who monitored my vital signs while inquiring about my status, and of course myself. My fear of flying disappeared completely as the intensity of the pain drowned all emotions. I lay still, not seeing or doing anything, not even thinking, just waiting for the landing.

This was not my first flight. It had been nineteen years since I had boarded an Eastern Airlines plane headed for the United States, disembarking in Baltimore, Maryland where Mr. and Mrs. George and their two children, the family with whom I would work and share a home, met me. It was night when I arrived on February 21, 1970. The scenery had changed from blue skies and white clouds above to a sea of artificial lights beneath the airplane. The weather had changed from tropical to a North American cold that made me reach for the coat I had brought with me.

The Georges recognized me from the photo I had sent to them when I was seeking a sponsor back in Jamaica. It was a blessing that such kind people had decided to sponsor me. They accepted me as a part of their family, giving me one of the four bedrooms upstairs next to the children's, welcoming me at their dinner table and taking me out to dinner at some of the finest restaurants with them. When I told them I liked going to church they found me a Methodist Church that I could attend. Although it was far from their home they gave me a ride to and from church every Sunday until I made friends who assumed the responsibility. I transferred my membership from the church in Jamaica and joined the ladies' duckpin bowling league. This helped to ease the pain of having to leave my own loving family, four younger sisters, Shirley, Georgia, LaVerne and AlvaJoy, two younger brothers, Harold and Hugh, my grandmother, Mammie, an only aunt, Aunt Lin, uncles and cousins.

My mother was already in America, living in Connecticut, and my father was working on a ship. I was a bit nervous about my future in a new country with a new job and new home, even flying for the first time but, being a precocious young woman at the age of twenty-three I was ready for this adventure. The adventure got more exciting after meeting the Georges who treated me kindly, but I still became home sick and cried for a few weeks while using most of my fifty dollars a week pay check for long distance phone bills to call home and friends in New York.

Sitting by a window on the plane I had watched until my homeland became a dot in the Caribbean Sea. The clouds welcomed me for the next few hours and the sun glistened off the wings of the airplane. As the plane soared higher and higher I swallowed harder and harder to prevent explosion of my eardrums from the cabin pressure. Now, on this copter I could not enjoy the scenery and felt no cabin pressure, only pain.

AT THOMAS JEFFERSON UNIVERSITY HOSPITAL

When we finally arrived at Thomas Jefferson Hospital, the same statement was made: no pain medication could be administered until the diagnosis was determined. Meanwhile, being log rolled from one stretcher to another caused the pain to intensify, and my pleas not to be moved went unheard. I vividly remember the doctor telling me that he had to put screws into the sides of my head and in my knees. Not understanding, I asked if this would affect my brain. He said they would not go in that far. I told him I wanted to discuss it with my husband, but I had no idea where Charley was. The doctor said there was no time to wait for Charley; it had to be done immediately. I was alone and scared in this sterile room, and did not trust this man claiming to be a doctor.

Finally they gave me some medication. Although medicated, I could still feel the screws being inserted into my head and knees. When my husband arrived (later I learned it was the following day), one look at me sent him into shock as he could not recognize the woman he had married. I could not imagine what I looked like. The sides of my head had been shaved to accommodate the screws that had been attached to some weights to stabilize my body. Not only was I encased by large pieces of metal, cords and wires, I was on an unconventional bed that rocked from side to side. He exclaimed, "Fay! What happened to you?" I asked where had he been, and told him how I had wanted to discuss it with him before they were put on, but the doctor had said I couldn't wait. He was tired, upset and frightened. He stayed with me that night until late, then retired to the hospital's dormitory, recommended to him by one of the nurses, at a cost of forty dollars per night. Later he told me of his ordeal to get to the hospital, the many times he had been lost and the hell he had gone through trying to find me.

For two and a half days I remained in this miserable, uncomfortable position. Whenever the bed tilted to either side, my body tensed in fear of falling. I mentioned my fear to one of the nurses, and it was at that moment that I learned I was strapped against the bed. However, this fact did not change my feelings or my fears and my body continued to tense whenever the bed tilted.

Early Tuesday morning, August 1, 1989, I was on the operating table. Would I survive this? I heard that the surgery lasted twelve and a half hours. Then followed blood transfusion, since the doctor said too much blood had been lost during the surgery. One incident that stands out in my mind is the doctor standing by my bed and saying, "You are a lucky woman." He said the damage was bad, but the surgery was a success, although he was not sure if many of the damaged nerves would return. He also mentioned that a lot of time had been spent removing bone fragments from my spinal cord. I am not sure when these statements were made; it could have been the day of the surgery or the morning after. Time was foggy to me. Since time was not clear I do not know how many days were spent in the Intensive Care Unit. I do remember being moved to another room, still in extreme pain, with many wires attached to my weak body, and hooked up to a self-administered morphine drip.

I continuously pressed the button of the self-administered morphine drip, but instead of relief came hallucinations, in which I saw the lights outside my window as men's faces, and when I slept, dreams were nightmares. I was in a Russian prison (why Russian I would never know) being tortured by the guards. Nurses who came to turn me were people trying to kill me. The experience was, to say the least, terrifying. I mentioned this to my sister Georgia on one of her visits. Being a nurse, she knew the side effects of the morphine and asked the doctors to replace it with pills. I felt much better, and my visitors also remarked that I looked better and conversed sensibly (I was not aware of my behavior while on the morphine) however, no pill could eliminate the pain.

The many doctors who visited early every morning had to be interns, because my main doctor, Dr. Cotter, who was always present, explained my diagnosis each morning and they would always be amazed. Being confined to lying on my sides or flat on my back created another problem.

My hiatus hernia, which I had been diagnosed with years earlier, prevented me from lying in a completely flat position and, although there were two pillows elevating my head, my bed still had to be set at an angle. Once the bed was set at a comfortable angle, I did not want it moved and argued with the nurses who wanted to lower it to change the sheets. For some reason it never felt as comfortable after resetting it.

With me being in Philadelphia and the kids in Connecticut, Charley traveled back and forth between both states. He had arranged for family to care for them. Our sister-in-law Tamsy, my sisters and my mother made sure they were fed and not alone. They were old enough to help themselves, at ages fourteen, twelve and nine so Charley laid out their clothes for school the previous night, then in the morning they dressed themselves and boarded the school bus that stopped in front of our driveway while he went to work. Charley said he had gone to the school and told the principal about the accident, and then he would call the school to ask if the children arrived safely.

A liquid diet had taken the place of the intravenous. Later, when I was introduced to solid food, I barely ate, mainly because it was hard to eat lying down and being fed. I could not read, and had no desire to watch television. Restricted by pain, my life was controlled by the nurses, who fed me, gave me sponge baths, turned me every few hours and handed me things from my bedside table which was impossible for me to reach, although it was so close. They also emptied the urinary bag that was attached to the Foley catheter which they had inserted in my bladder because I was unable to pass my own urine. Once the Foley was removed the nurses had to insert a urinary catheter every four hours to remove my urine.

One day I had a dreadful experience. My bladder felt like it was about to explode, the pain in my back was at its highest level, and my head became dizzy. There was no one available to catch me. Why was I being tortured? I asked myself, as I continued to press the call button. The torture continued another day when my body was fully inserted, with the exception of my head, into a big round machine. I had to lie still in the same position while they were doing the test. It could have been only half an hour, but being in extreme pain and unable to move gave me the sensation of being trapped in an underground mine for many hours. Even though my head was not covered, I felt as if I was going to suffocate. I don't know if it was a "CAT

Scan" or a "MRI" but this was the worst test I had ever taken. That day remains one of my most unforgettable days.

Slowly, during my recovery, I gathered this information about my injury: my back was broken, my two splintered vertebrae stuck into my spinal cord. The covering of my spinal cord was torn exposing the nerves and several nerves were damaged. My level of injury was L2 with spinal fusion from L1 through L4, and my spine was also cracked (a friend told me the doctor had compared my damage to that of someone crushing a Styrofoam cup in their hand). The doctors had cut my hip-bone and used it to fuse the two broken vertebrae. A metal rod held by large screws had been inserted into my back. This metal rod would prevent me from taking the important test called "MRI." (This I learned years later when I was required to take a MRI). My chances of walking again were questionable.

Four months later when I was about to leave the rehabilitation hospital I learned that I would never be able to urinate and defecate normally again. The loss of sensation in certain areas of my body would be permanent. Changes in my lifestyle would include not being able to lift, bend, do long standing, sitting, walking, and dancing. Medication and a special diet would become routine forever. Slowly I learned the steps I had to take towards my recovery. I would leave the hospital in a full body cast to rehabilitate in a nursing home.

On August 7th, 1989, an assistant pushed my stretcher to a special room which had two metal rails and a chain hanging from above. My memory fails to recall the exact number of men who were present, either five or six. One of the men instructed me to hold on with both hands to the chain. In my birthday suit, with legs held wide apart, I hung in mid air while they briskly wrapped my naked body from my breast to my knees, with the material that was becoming a cast. The area around the vagina and the rectum was left open for obvious reasons. Given the option to choose the color, I chose yellow, my favorite color. Yellow reminded me of the sun, which gives me energy. Maybe it would help to brighten the dark days ahead. The cast had to be dried onto my body, so it was left with rough edges that stuck into my arms and legs, while the rest of my body itched. This caused great discomfort and I was in hell. I imagined the warmth of the yellow melting the rough edges poking into my skin and soothing the itch.

The next day, they took me to another work- room where a different man cut another hole in the stomach area and lined all rough edges with a soft cloth. He then nailed a narrow strip of board across my thighs, preventing my legs from closing. When I learned from the doctor that this cell was to be my home for the next four months, I was devastated, and almost went crazy.

As confined as my body was, my mind had to expand. I realized that I had taken life for granted, my activities, work, family and home. Looking back over my life, I saw myself growing up in Jamaica, an island that I consider a paradise. Growing up at a time that we refer to as the "good old days," when mom bought fresh meat from the butcher's shop and the milkman delivered fresh milk straight from the cows' udders to our doors; so fresh it had to be scalded before use. Later we used the rich cream that gathered on the top to make butter. Likewise freshly baked bread was brought on horse drawn carriages from the bakery.

Tourism was one of Jamaica's most lucrative businesses and tourists yearned to bask in the hot golden sun on the white sand beaches, swim in the Caribbean

Sea that reflected the blue of the skies above it, relax under a huge tree, relishing the cool breeze and sipping a glass of the Island's famous rum punch. They enjoyed a variety of the spicy foods that awakened their taste buds such as Curried Goat, Ackee with Codfish (Ackee is a fleshy fruit from Africa that is grown in the Caribbean), and Escovitched fresh fish (various seasonings sautéed in oil and vinegar, then poured over fried fish).

One could also choose from a variety of fresh fruits grown throughout the Island. Mangoes, Oranges, Water Coconut, Sweet Sop and Jackfruit are just a handful of the many fruits that could be found in the hotels, the markets, on roadside stands being sold by vendors and hanging from the trees. Actually every tree in Jamaica bears something that can be eaten. I always said no one could die from hunger there.

The tropical weather allows hundreds of different species of flowers to bloom continuously throughout the year, creating breath-taking scenery all around the Island. It's possible that the warm weather could have contributed to the characteristics of the people: happy, friendly and fun loving. Regardless of how poor they were they knew how to laugh and party. Entertainment included telling stories, playing games such as hide and seek, dominos, and bingo; going to Saturday night dances, and Tuesday night triple bill. There were no televisions then; that came later.

In December the evening breeze is chilly enough for a sweater. It's relaxing, romantic and everyone looks forward to celebrating Christmas. When my American friend asked me if we celebrate Christmas in Jamaica, I laughed then replied, "Your celebration doesn't compare to ours." We celebrate for three days starting from Christmas Eve when the sounds of firecrackers outdo the sound of the Reggae music. Outside children display their starlight while mothers bake Plum Pudding, Christmas cookies and make our special drinks called Sorrel, Ginger Beer and Rum Punch. We do a thorough cleaning of our houses and replace old curtains and bedspreads with new ones, then decorate the Christmas tree. The trees outside are also lighted and decorated.

Some people attend church on Christmas day in new dresses made just for that day. One thing that stands out in my mind is waking up early Christmas morning to the sweet singing of the carolers, and then going to Christmas market with my mother. All the stores are closed, the streets are blocked downtown and vendors spread toys and gifts all over the streets creating what is called a "Christmas Market." On our way home we are greeted by the "Junkanoos," who are men dressed in costumes and masks doing their traditional dance with its roots in Africa, to the beat of their drums, fifes and other instruments. I was very afraid of them although I knew they were men under the costumes.

Of course we also have Santa Claus, who we called Father Christmas. After opening our gifts, as children, we enjoyed a special breakfast of fresh fruits, coffee, hard dough bread, Ackee with codfish and fried dumplings. The day after Christmas is called "Boxing Day" that's when the real partying occurs, with dancing and visiting friends and family. This is my favorite holiday.

Always having the basic necessities of life, food, shelter, clothing and a loving family, I was not poverty-stricken. With my mother's motto of "Good better best, never let it rest until your good is better and your better is best," we moved to many different homes in search of the best. At each home, events occurred that left a lasting memory with me. The first home I recall living in, I was about six years old, but I remember that the floor of the small place my parents rented was so shine it could almost be used as a mirror. In one corner of the bedroom nicely displayed like another room was my doll's furniture; dresser, table, chairs, cabinet filled with china, and a bed so big my sister was often laid on it when she was a baby. At the second home, three of us moved in but soon there were four, my second sister Shirley was delivered in my mother's bedroom, delivered by a midwife six years after I was born.

When I was about seven years old a chain of accidents started at that house that would last a lifetime. Only now do I realize that I am "accident-prone." The first accident happened when I climbed on a high stool to pick flowers, suddenly as if someone had pushed me I fell off the stool hitting the back of my head causing an open wound that left a scar. Shortly after that incident, I was sitting at the kitchen table waiting to have a cup of hot cocoa that my father was preparing. The pot of hot, dark, sweet drink spilled making its way down my left hip leaving another scar on my body.

Later we moved to my maternal grandmother's place. It was in what we called a tenement yard, with many rooms rented to different people. I remember the huge grape arbor at the front of the yard and the pit toilet which scared me with its dark, gaping hole. On most Saturday nights they would hold dances next door and, being too young to attend, I would stand at the fence and watch the people dance. Maybe that's where my love of dancing started. This yard was also where my most haunting experience took place.

The little shop at the front of the property was my father's first business; he started a bakery and pastry shop. He delivered his baked buns, patties, hard-dough bread and other pastries to the small area businesses while selling some in the shop. He also worked as a policeman before he started working on a ship. We did not see him for months at a time, but when he came home he brought us lots of goodies from his travels around the world. Once he brought me a doll the size of a newborn baby with skin as soft as a human's; she was programmed to talk and showed two teeth as if she was smiling. Mom said the custom's fees for the doll cost more than the mattress he brought in at the same time.

Being the first child, I was spoiled with lots of toys and clothes. My mother made me pretty dresses from fabric she bought by the pound. She would sew me a dress in one night. That was when she taught me to do the

27

"handwork", that is, hem, base and put in zippers. I also learned the different types of fabric; linen, cotton, nylon and taffeta by helping her. At Christmas and Easter I got two new dresses, seldom did I wear the same dress twice to church. I was brought back to the reality of being in the hospital when the therapist appeared to do therapy on my legs.

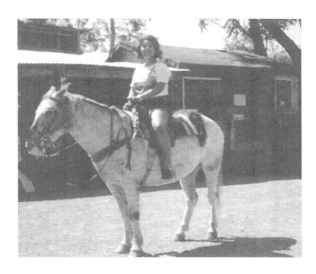

Figure 1: Fay and Toby at the stables

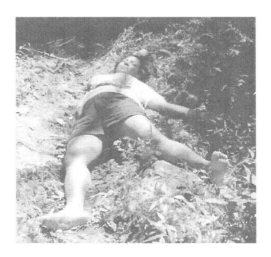

Figure 2: On the path after the fall

29

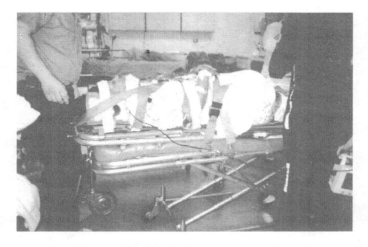

Figure 3: Fay and the emergency team

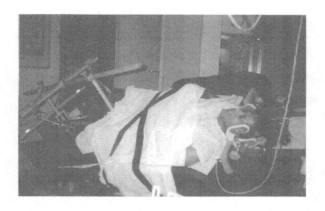

Figure 4: In traction

CHAPTER 2

LIFE IN A BODY CAST

W ith the cast on, I could do nothing but lie in bed and wait for my back to heal. Therapists gave me physical therapy on my arms, legs and feet daily. They tied a therapeutic band to the side of my bed and told me to pull on it as often as I could to exercise my arms.

It was about that time that I started helping myself by brushing my teeth and giving my upper body a sponge bath while a nurse held the basin of water. I could not reach my lower body, which the nurses continued to sponge. Feeding myself was not hard, since my appetite still had not returned. The food always went back after I had picked at it.

Medications continued throughout the day; for pain, which was incessant, for the stomach, because I was lying down constantly, and stool softeners and blood thinner to prevent clots since I was inactive. The latter, called

31

Heparin was administered in the form of an injection directly below my navel twice a day. I was scared to death of the needle although it was small, and never got accustomed to it, even after three months. My body still rocks with fear when I think about it being inserted in this most sensitive area, which never lost sensation. Usually injections are given in the derriere; unfortunately, since I lost sensation there, I got it in my belly where I had sensation.

I pressed the call button whenever I needed to be turned. This took two people. If only one was available I would have to wait until another was on hand to help. Pillows were an important aid in my recovery. They helped to keep me on my side, while supporting my back and my leg that hung in mid air due to the board across the cast. These pillows had to be removed and restocked properly each time I was turned.

With my life on hold, awaiting the healing process, I could not stay in the hospital. Without my knowledge the doctors had decided to put me in a nursing home in Philadelphia.

FAMILY AND FRIENDS

I was locked in my own little world of pain and misery, thoughtless of how my family, relatives, and friends were feeling. It wasn't until they started calling and visiting that I realized their pain. I did not know when Charley had called to tell them about the accident. I understand they were all upset that such an unkind fate should befall their beloved family member: sister, daughter, and mother.

They started praying immediately for my recovery, between their tears and mental anguish. They traveled from Connecticut to Philadelphia to see me. I will always remember the first day my mother saw me; she whispered to my husband that I had moved my leg. I pretended not to hear, and wondered why she was so amazed, not knowing that they were worried about me not walking again. They all knew how Fay loved to dance. Their love and support would be among the medications to help bring me through the rough times ahead. I did not know this at the time.

The news had spread and people were calling from everywhere: my job, my neighbors, friends and relatives. I had planned on telling many people about my horseback riding experience, how wonderful it had been, before the accident. I never realized from the huge network of family and friends I had how many would actually hear about it.

During one of his calls home, Charley had learned from one of his brothers that he had family living in Philadelphia, close to the hospital. This happened to be his brother-in-law, Johnny, and his wife Minnette. What a blessing for Charley and me. They visited every night, bringing me home-cooked meals. Minnette fed, washed and lotioned me. When it wasn't possible for both, one came. Their generous accommodation of Charley in their home not only saved him hotel costs; it also saved him from going insane. Being so far from home and meeting such good people to help in a tragedy was a miracle.

The fact that my children had had to be picked up on their return from camp had completely left my mind. When my sister Georgia had met them on their arrival from camp, she did not tell them about the accident. She thought it would be better for their father to do so. I understand that when he did, they did not believe him and looked into closets while telling him to stop joking. When my daughter realized it was not a joke she started crying. Later, she confessed to me that she had suspected something was wrong when she did not see me waiting at the bus stop to pick them up like I had been doing for the past years. Then my son Sean told me that he said, "Something is wrong because Mom always came to pick us up."

My two younger sisters, Georgia and Shirley, who are nurses, questioned the doctors about my prognosis, and when they were told of the plan to transfer me into a nursing home, they told the doctors they would have me transferred to Gaylord Rehabilitation Hospital in Wallingford, Connecticut.

My sisters made many long distance calls to Gaylord, to me and to the social workers at Jefferson Hospital. I was not aware of the problems my sisters had arranging my transfer. They had to arrange for my admittance to Gaylord, and transportation to get me there. Gaylord was known as one of the best rehabilitation hospitals in the country and I felt lucky to be accepted, and blessed that there was a vacant room awaiting my arrival.

My stay in Jefferson Hospital was approximately two weeks. On August 14, 1989, excited to be going close to home, it was not hard to say goodbye to the nurses, doctors and therapists when it was time for them to put my stretcher into the ambulance that was to transport me to the airport to board the helicopter for Gaylord Rehabilitation Hospital.

The beauty of the day almost rivaled the day the accident had occurred. As the ambulance sped through the streets of Philadelphia, I noticed there were no sirens this time; the emergency was over. After two weeks in the hospital room, it was a pleasure to see the skies without having to look through a hospital window, although having to lie on my back allowed me a view of only the top of trees and tall buildings. At the small airport, again two men lifted my stretcher onto the air ambulance. The three people aboard were the pilot, a courteous nurse and myself.

The flight was almost enjoyable since I wasn't in the intense pain I had been in when being flown from the Pocono Hospital to the Jefferson Hospital. Thank God and the doctors for painkillers. On arrival in Connecticut, another quiet ambulance drove me to Gaylord Hospital. Gaylord welcomed me like they just knew I was some beloved relative who had finally returned home. My mother, Urceline, and my sister Georgia, who awaited my arrival, supplied the front desk with the necessary information while someone pushed me to my room. My husband and children visited later that evening.

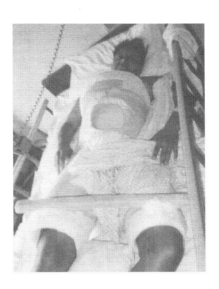

Figure 5: In body cast

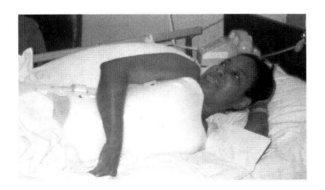

Figure 6: In body jacket

CHAPTER 3

LIFE AT GAYLORD

S ituated in a tranquil country setting in Wallingford, Connecticut, Gaylord looked like a vacation cottage. A small hospital with only two floors, it is an adult rehabilitation hospital that helps people with traumatic brain injury, stroke and spinal cord injury, to return to a life style that is as normal as possible. Physical and occupational therapy is given to all the patients, and support is given to family members. This helped my husband to cope better with my tragedy.

I immediately felt some comfort at Gaylord, which was good since this would be my home for the next four months. Room number 208 was now mine, private, immaculate, with a big picture window which gave me an expansive view of the well manicured lawns and countless trees. Mounted on one wall was a painting (I believe it was of water rushing against the rocks), and a large bulletin board, a clock and a small television in the corner. On another wall, there were shelves, stacked with catheters and supplies that I would be using. Next to the shelves sat a counter with a sink, and the mirror over the sink showed a reflection of the room. Around the corner was a bathroom, which I would not be able to use for three months. There were two chairs to accommodate my visitors, one bedside table, a tray table on which my meals were served, and above my bed was the famous call button, my only link to survival.

After I was settled in bed, I was offered lunch. For the first time I could say I enjoyed my sandwich more than any food I had received at the other hospital. I felt more relaxed, as if I was home. Shortly after lunch the medical doctor introduced herself. Her name was Dr. Lacey. The urologist, orthopedist, psychiatrist, physiatrist, and the social worker came later. Joining the group were different nurses, therapists, and a priest. They all marveled at my cast. Some had read about it, and informed me that it was called a "Spic Cast" and had been used in hospitals years ago.

Dr. Murray, the orthopedist, visited only once a month so it was a few weeks before we met. I had hoped that his verdict on the length of my stay in the body cast would be different, but he confirmed what the other doctor had said. For the first time since the accident my tears started to flow. When he said, "Yes, it is four months," my emotions broke to pieces just like my back had. In my mind's eyes, four months was four years. I could not perceive how an active person like me would survive in that bed, in that cast, that long. As the tears streamed down, the doctor held my hand and said with pity, "I am sorry, I wish I could help."

Depression set in for a while. Some days I came close to insanity. At times I had a great urge to get up and walk, but had to dismiss the thought before I made any movement. I often wonder where I would be without the help of prayer, visitors, and the television. Among the gifts I had received were some books, including another book on Spinal Cord Injury from Gaylord, (the other hospital had given me one) but I could neither concentrate on reading nor find a comfortable position to hold a book. It was the homely atmosphere, hospitable medical staff and the friendly therapists who worked on my arms and legs that helped me adjust to my situation in my new "home." I fell in love with the place and the staff.

Initially, the treatment there was similar to that at

Jefferson Hospital; the Heparin injection below my navel, the medications, doctor's visits, the cathing, changing my position every three to four hours, and the therapeutic band tied to the bed. However, as I progressed, therapy increased.

A typical day at Gaylord started at 7 a.m. with brushing my teeth, eating breakfast, a sponge bath to the open areas around the cast, and changing the bed. What a chore it was to change that bed. The many pillows that aided in my recovery had to be changed, and my body had to be log rolled from side to side as they replaced the dirty sheets with clean ones. The few private hours I had until 11 a.m., when my therapist arrived to work on my arms, were spent watching television. Lunch followed shortly after, and by 2 p.m. my favorite therapist, Deena, worked on my legs and feet.

Deena worked with me throughout my stay there, and finally got me walking in the fourth month. We had so much fun together, I am sure she was a part of my cure. I looked forward to therapy with Deena even as it got harder to do. Between pain and therapy was laughter and chatting. One of our most outrageous moments was when she told me that her husband said to her, "You are such a hemorrhoid." We almost died with laughter. Having experienced hemorrhoids when I was pregnant, I knew how ugly and painful they could be. This convinced me that that was the worst name he could have called her.

After Deena left, I watched television until dinner was served. In the evenings I had visitors. At nights, I was given another sponge bath. Then followed the bowel program which I hated because in this program, the nurse inserted a suppository into my rectum where it stayed for about half an hour before she manually removed the feces from my bowels. Again, the television was my companion until I fell asleep. Some nights I slept well, some nights I didn't.

The ritual of waking me to be catheterized at three every morning bothered me, because sometimes I could not go back to sleep and by 7 a.m. I would have to be up whether I wanted to sleep or not. There were good days when I had no problems and bad days when I was very sick. Urinary tract infections were many, and the medications used to treat them started a chain of reactions. My stomach became upset, which caused vomiting, followed by yeast infection. The nurses told me to drink lots of water and cranberry juice, this produced too much urine, and since I had to be catheterized, my fluid intake had to be moderate. Reason being, cathing time would be more often and it is not good to be introducing something foreign into the bladder too often, as it causes infections. When an infection was not present, constipation was. The inability to defecate made me very ill; the medication for this triggered diarrhea, and then the nurses' job increased by having to change my sheets continuously along with cleaning my body. At this point, therapy had to be cancelled.

Therapy was on Mondays through Fridays, but the weekends were free. After a few weeks of therapy in my room, it was time to change the scenery and to mingle with other patients and therapists, so the nurses' log rolled me onto a stretcher and pushed me to the gym every afternoon. I was amazed by the number of disabled people scattered around the gym, working from wheelchairs, mats, stationary bikes, walkers, weight benches and learning the board transfer (method of moving from wheelchair to another seat, e.g. car or bed, and vice versa, by sliding on a board). I was the only one on a stretcher, but it was exciting to be among other people after being in seclusion. A few would be leaving for home the following week. The Central Park jogger, (the woman who was raped and beaten while jogging in Central Park) whom I had heard was also a patient there at the time would be leaving in a few days. I envied them and wondered when my turn would come, since it was indefinite.

My new therapist Tim started me lifting one-pound weights and rapidly increased it to twenty-five pounds. Lying on my back in the cast, I found this difficult and I cried, "I can't do it," while he laughingly replied, "Come on, you can do it." On beautiful days patients were pushed outside to enjoy the outdoors and to do therapy. I still have vivid memories of Deena and me under the tree having fun while building muscles. When I wasn't doing therapy I would lie outside and watch the others ride around in their wheelchairs, while nurses smoked on their break time. I longed for the day when I would be sitting in a wheelchair.

AM I LUCKY?

While I lay in the rehabilitation hospital waiting for my back to heal, friends and relatives visiting exclaimed how lucky I was. Confined and in pain, I could not understand why they thought I was lucky. My thoughts flashed back to the doctor in Philadelphia who had performed the surgery. Looking seriously into my face, he was the first to remark, "You are a lucky woman." I was unable to comprehend his statement then. Although the incident remained in my mind, the words were not significant. One gorgeous Sunday afternoon, as my husband Charley visited, he said, "Fay, you are lucky." It was then that I replied to the remark, "I fell off a horse and broke my back and you think I am lucky?" He answered, "You are alive." True, I was alive, but my human nature saw only the negative things.

Lying there for four months was only a part of my problem. I had to wait for someone, regardless of age, color or sex, to do absolutely everything for me, including emptying my bladder and bowels, washing me and changing my positions. Different reasons were given for being lucky: "It could have been your head on that rock, and your spinal cord could have been severed," however, "You are alive" was most common. I do not consider myself lucky because I escaped death at that point. I am still going to die; it was not yet time. When someone is the victim of a life-threatening accident but not killed, I believe timing rather than "luck" determines the outcome. It's the opinion of many people that regardless of one's condition he or she is lucky to be alive. My belief is that it doesn't make sense to be alive and not living.

Still, like a broken record, the words "You are lucky" were said to me daily. I wondered if people knew the meaning of "lucky." One dictionary defines the word as "having good fortune, producing or resulting in good by chance, favorable." None of these meanings applied to me! I did not win the lottery; neither did an old uncle die leaving me a fortune. Where the hell was the luck?

I began to understand a few weeks later when I was pushed on a stretcher to the solarium for a change of environment. The interaction with other accident victims opened my eyes to the reality. The first patient who introduced himself told me how long he had been there and said his family had visited him earlier in his calamity but no longer came and seldom called.

In contrast, my friends and family visited every day. They brought gifts, flowers, food, expressions of love, and words of encouragement. Even the bulletin board was jammed with cards, each of which made me feel special. Some of those cards came from my children's classmates, whose teachers allowed them time from their class work for the project (see Appendix). I was so touched, I cried. One nurse asked if I was a teacher. After hearing how I got the cards, she said, "Oh I would cry." I replied, "I did." Some co-workers made donations for me, and two of them wrote an inspiring article in the department's magazine. Churches of all denominations in London, Jamaica, and the United States of America were praying for my recovery without even meeting me. After I returned home an acquaintance exclaimed, "Oh you are the person my church was praying for!" Her minister was asked by a friend of mine to pray for me.

So many cared; some took the time to just sit with me, watching television, talking and praying. Others accompanied me to the gym and waited while I did my therapy. My friends who resided in New York had traveled by train and car to visit me. The ones who could not visit called from places like London, Jamaica, Florida and Texas. One particular friend, Mr. Clark, took the train and walked a few miles to the hospital, because he did not have a ride. Another friend was surprised when she saw my plants and flowers crowded together on the windowsill. Still holding her Mum plant, she remarked, "I was thinking that this may be the only plant you will have, but you have so much there is no room for this." That windowsill and my table so full of plants, flowers, fruits, and gifts affirmed how my people felt about me. Their display of love was comforting and reassuring. Now I could appreciate their efforts and the outpouring of deep concern and real affection overwhelmed me.

More good fortune too, in that two of my sisters are nurses and gave me physical as well as personal support. Arranging for my admittance to Gaylord and preventing my being sent to a nursing home was only the beginning of their love and support. Sister Georgia kept my body in good condition by washing me then applying lotion to prevent dry skin, while Sister Shirley dutifully did my laundry daily, even after working all night. Sometimes she fell asleep waiting for it to finish. Luckily she did not fall asleep while driving to the hospital, because she always took the longer journey of the back roads since she is not a highway driver. Sister LaVerne was my beautician; she kept my finger and toenails manicured, and helped Georgia to wash my hair. The special body oils and lotions brought in by my sister-in-law Cynthia, from her line of cosmetics, "Cyntay Cosmetics" helped enormously in removing the dead skin and dryness. My sister-in law Tamsy helped at home with my children when she wasn't visiting, bringing a gift each visit. Brother Harold brought in a VCR and movies for me. (The week I was leaving I discovered that the hospital provided this service.) My mother, husband, and my children were always there, doing whatever they could to make me happy.

My birthday in the hospital was the best. I anxiously awaited the orthopedist's monthly visit that day, thinking the best present I could get was to be told I would be free of the cast. I was overjoyed when he said, "I think you can get out of this cast now." The doctor in Philadelphia had said four months before it could be removed, and it was only two and a half months. I could only lie there and thank God. This alone would have been enough gift, but that night, my niece Kay and her husband Ruddy sent a clown with balloons, in the middle of the surprise party my mother had planned. The nurse had said I would be attending a meeting on spinal cord injury as she pushed my bed to the solarium. Shocked but happy to see my family in this fully decorated place with so much food, I realized this was in my honor, and I was stunned. My only regret was not being able to sit up and enjoy eating my big

Taylor

stuffed lobster, because lying down made the food less palatable.

I also realized how lucky I was in other areas that my family and friends didn't. For nine years my husband and I had two health insurances. In 1988 our tax person advised us to cancel one, saying it did not make sense having two. I cancelled mine, and had my accident in 1989. I was extremely upset that I had listened to her. Nevertheless, I was lucky that I had an insurance to cover some of my medical bills. "Long term disability" had been just words on paper. Not once did it ever occur to me that I would need it. I was lucky though, that my company offered it, because I am unable to work due to pain, bowel and bladder dysfunction, and sitting for long periods of time becomes unbearable. Still unable to walk long distance, I rely on a straight cane. Thank God long-term disability existed.

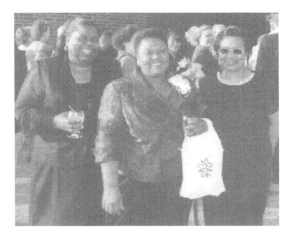

Figure 7: Georgia, Shirley and Fay

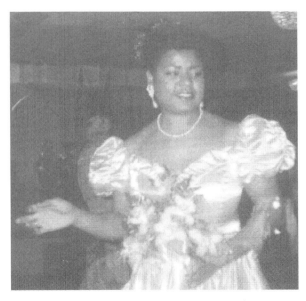

Figure 8: Sister AlvaJoy/Joy/Babylin

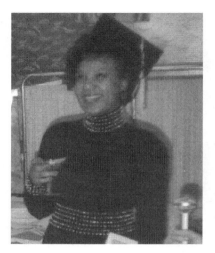

Figure 9: LaVerne

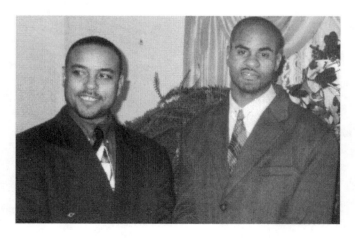

Figure 10: brothers Hugh and Harold

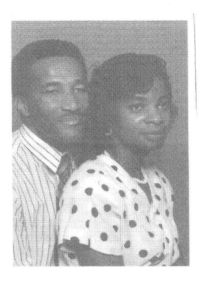

Figure 11: Johnny and Minnette

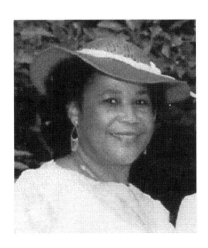

Figure 12: Tamsy

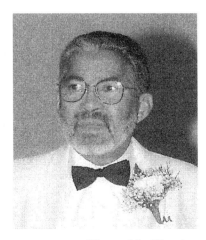

Figure 13: Norris

53

CHAPTER 4

MOVING TOWARDS RECOVERY

T hree months in bed seemed like three years. I watched the seasons change from my window and thought of myself as a turtle in a shell. But finally a body jacket replaced my cast. The day the cast was removed, Friday October 20th, was another day of torture. I lay there powerless, breathless, never ceasing to pray as the man ran the noisy electric saw close to my feeble body. With every cut into the rock- hard material my heart slipped into my mouth, while my nerves shook from the annoying noise.

Since my body jacket was not ready, a temporary one was made from the cast. This was very uncomfortable because the sides were taped around my torso and it often became uneven. Although it was not perfect, it allowed me to turn myself. I held onto the bed rail with my hands, placed one foot firmly on the bed then threw my body over to my side. I wanted to keep it a secret that the cast was cut off, and surprise my family on their next visit, but I couldn't. I still remember my husband's ecstasy when I told him on the phone.

One week later, on Friday October 27th, I received my permanent body jacket, which I would have to wear for another four months. My reward was a wheelchair! I could not sit upright immediately since I had been lying down for such a long time, so a therapist put me into a position between sitting and lying, an extremely uncomfortable position. A few days later, Deena, my therapist, slowly brought me to a sitting position an inch at a time while monitoring my blood pressure as I sat upright. The ability to sit up made my day. For my son Sean, I was now a big toy with whom he took pleasure in giving zooming rides around the hospital on his Sunday visits. With fear of crashing I would yell "Slow down!" To celebrate, my brother -in-law, Norris, performed a calypso concert for all the patients. We gathered in the lounge, moving our heads to the music, forgetting our wheelchairs for a while.

Along with this promotion came retraining. A nurse had told me that when the cast came off, my vacation would be over. She was right. Therapy increased from two to four times a day, then to five. I had to re-learn everything, including potty training, and crawling before walking. I had felt pressured when the weights rapidly increased from two to twenty five pounds lying on my back. Now the words "P.T." meant "Pain and Torture" instead of physical therapy, and my screams echoed as my hamstrings were stretched.

A typical day now was as follows: up at seven, breakfast at seven thirty, a sponge bath at eight, physical therapy at nine thirty with Deena, occupational therapy at ten and ten thirty, physical therapy at eleven thirty a.m. with Deena, lunch at twelve p.m., physical therapy at two p.m. with Tim, and at two thirty with Carl, another friendly young man. By the time I returned to my room at three p.m. exhaustion had taken over my body. I rested until four thirty when dinner was served. Sometimes I waited in the solarium where I conversed with other patients about our accidents, and emotions, past and present.

I learnt to wheel myself around the hospital and outdoors. One morning as I wheeled down the hallway, I saw a man with a tracheotomy. This brought back memories of my co-worker Sly, whose car had slipped off a ramp while he was underneath fixing it in 1983. He was paralyzed from his neck down and stayed on the same floor in the same hospital. With pain in my heart I had visited him, not knowing I also would be there. Remembering Sly, I felt blessed, because I could breathe without a tracheotomy, and my hands were mobile so I could somewhat help myself.

At therapy, a few days after those pitiful thoughts of Sly, I noticed a sad-looking young man next to me doing his therapy better than me. I wished I could have pulled the stiff band with as much strength. After he left, I mentioned my observations to the therapist, who said, "He is paralyzed." Mixed feelings of shock, pity and anger encompassed my body. Why did this happen to such a young handsome man, with such a gorgeous body? In comparison to him I was lucky, because I was older, already had a family and most important would walk again.

The first time on my feet, I understood how the months of weight lifting had prepared me for that day. My now strong arms supported my body and allowed me to move my feet. Soon after starting between two rails, I went to a walker. Weeks later, I graduated to two prong canes and finally a straight cane. Years after learning to walk, I still relied on my wheelchair, because I was not strong enough to walk long distances. When I discovered the joy of walking again, I left my wheelchair when I was alone in my room and watered my plants on the windowsill. I felt fulfilled doing something meaningful. My plants were one of the important things in my life. I have always loved plants. As a child the plants in the yard were my friends to whom I spoke after school and I have had plants everywhere I live.

During my walks with Deena, we went to almost every corner of the hospital, at the same time practicing climbing the stairs. It was not hard to climb these steps since I had been practicing on the stairs that were made for therapy in the gym. However, I still had to put both feet on one step before moving to the next step.

I enjoyed the beauty of the greenhouse which made me feel elated, and I viewed the gift shop as we passed by. One of the most interesting places at Gaylord is called "Easy Street." It's a mini supermarket and restaurant with a parked car. Here patients learn how to cope with the outside world after rehabilitation. It was in that parked car that I learned to do my board transfer from wheelchair to car and vice versa. This is the method where a piece of board is placed between the wheelchair and the other seat (car, bed or whatever) and you slide across to get from one to the other. To complete the board transfer was a great accomplishment. I was one step ahead of helping myself. The following day when the nurse started to call for help to lift me to the bed, I told her to allow me to do the transfer. She was shocked but happy that I did it so easily. That was the start of my independence and they no longer had to lift me.

After three and a half months, I was allowed to spend one night at home to see how I would cope with my new condition. The caregivers held meetings with my family to discuss how I would manage and whether the bathroom was handicap-accessible. The stairs were the biggest concern; there was talk of rearranging the house. However I did so well, nothing had to be changed, except for the purchase of a commode, which doubled as a seat over the toilet and a shower chair.

The excitement started as I slid across the board from the wheelchair onto the seat of my car. No coke, heroin or crack could have given me the high that I felt that night driving home from the hospital. Seeing the streets, houses, lights along the way, and feeling the fresh night air, I realized then that I had forgotten about the real world.

Without my knowledge Charley had invited many friends and family members to welcome me. Having to entertain so many people was very tiring, but I could not complain, I thoroughly enjoyed the company. It felt great to be home after such a long time and to have people to share the joy with me. Some brought flowers and gifts. I was just learning to walk with the walker and each person wanted to see me walk, like a baby taking that first step. Their joyous faces showed the happiness they felt for me. Walking was easy. Self-catheterization (method of emptying the bladder) at home seemed impossible, but with pillows and my daughter Monique's help I was able to accomplish it that first night.

My brain draws a blank about the following morning, remembering only my happiness on returning to Gaylord. One secret fear that haunted me was the uncertainty of taking care of myself at home. I had grown accustomed to the nurses serving me and caring for me. The occupational therapist had been preparing me to be independent for my permanent stay at home. Simple things like fixing a sandwich, doing my laundry, and driving had to be re-learned, and the more difficult things like cathing and emptying my bowels had to be learned before leaving the hospital. When the therapist gave me a long round stick with an "S" shape on one end and a hook on the other, to help me reach things, I laughed and thought it was a stupid idea. It became an important helper in my life. I used it to remove clothes from the dryer, take sweaters from the shelf in the closet and was amazed at how well the contraption worked when putting on my pants and socks. I am glad I decided to give the little stick a try.

My first night at home went well, so the following week they allowed me to spend another day at home. These short trips were preparing me for my discharge. This time my sister Shirley picked me up and we stopped to buy some gifts for my favorite nurses. In my mind I felt normal, but my body was years away from normality. While shopping my body went into temporary paralysis. Realizing that I was not as strong as I thought, faster than lightning, I had to find an object to lean on, waiting there until Shirley finished the shopping. Fear of leaving the store filled my very soul: how would I walk back to the car? I felt too weak to move from where I stood. Shirley actually carried me to the car, while leaning on her we moved at a snail's pace to our destination.

HOME

Home.... this time permanently. The place I had longed to be, I felt like a stranger to. I had left on July 28th, 1989 and returned on November 29, 1989. It was good to be home; however I still had to look forward to continued therapy at Easter Seals Rehabilitation Center, visits to my medical doctor, the urologist, Gaylord outpatient clinic, and attending Spinal Cord Support Group at Newington Children's Hospital.

I immediately tried to get back to my normal life, but it was impossible. I was still weak, and almost passed out when I tried to clean the bathroom mirror. When grocery shopping, someone pushed me in the wheelchair because walking weakened me halfway through the store. Three years later when I thought I was strong enough to shop without the wheelchair I had to leave the store before I finished my shopping because of the weakness. This aggravated me because I would have to return another day to finish the shopping.

My outward appearance was remarkable. I kept myself looking beautiful, well dressed, hair nicely done, and some make-up so no one was aware of what I was enduring: the constant back pain, the weakness, the bladder and bowel discomfort, trying to keep track of the cathing times and having to wait for someone to lift my left leg, which still refused to respond.

My family and friends continued to visit, call and help. Sister Georgia took me to my doctors' appointments, sister Shirley cleaned my kitchen floor; a friend ironed our clothes, another friend helped with the gardening, and brother Hugh chauffeured me around. My husband had the ordeal of bathing me; since I was still wearing the body jacket (which I continued to wear for four months); a simple shower became a task. The T-shirt under the jacket had to be removed, and the jacket (in which I showered) replaced, then, removing the wet jacket, he dried both my body and the jacket, put on a clean T-shirt and replaced the dry jacket again. This process required my body to be log rolled on the bed repeatedly.

My children, Charles Jr., Sean and Monique, took turns dressing me before leaving for school. This meant rising earlier. One month later, my sister AlvaJoy arranged for home help. Being an independent person, it wasn't long before learning to buckle myself into the brace became easy by rolling from side to side on the bed. The stick with the "S" shape and the hook on the ends that the

Taylor

therapist had given me at Gaylord was used continuously, to put on my socks, pants and to reach things in high or low places. Sometimes I went down on my knees to reach things on the floor. I also figured how to use my feet to lotion my legs. These things were done naturally, because I was not able to bend normally. I told everyone that I would learn to bend during therapy, but when my therapist told me that the rod in my back would prevent me from bending normally that was another shock to me.

The numbness in my buttocks and thighs seemed to be gone; it had been seven years since the accident, but when the ice cream I was eating fell on my thigh, and I did not feel the coldness, I realized that I had grown accustomed to my new body that had no sensation, which was now normal for me. This was my initial life at home after my disability.

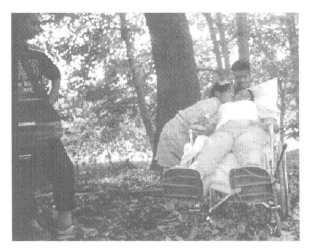

Figure 14: Fay and family in the woods

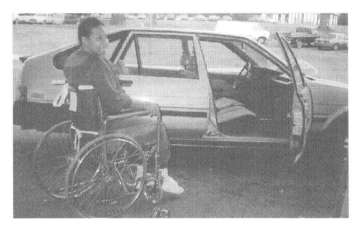

Figure 15: Going Home

CHAPTER 5

HUSBAND

W hen two people are joined together in Holy matrimony, a part of the vow says, "For better, for worse." The words are taken for granted with no thought of anything tragic happening in the marriage. I can only imagine what my husband must have experienced during this period. He must have felt as much pain as I did, watching me suffer, and handling a sudden increased work schedule. He still had to go to work; we needed money now more than ever. Added to his regular job was: cooking, laundry, writing the bills, caring for our children and giving me support.

The drive to visit me in the hospital was far and tiring. It involved many trips because I was there for a long time. The social worker told him that he should not feel guilty if he could not visit every day since there was nothing he could do to help me, instead a phone call would be just as good. He felt relieved and began calling more and visiting less. He became so lonely from my absence at home that he started a home study course. My return home was made easier in terms of his traveling to the hospital, but there were more responsibilities for him because I still needed help and could not offer my help around the house. Like one of the children I waited to be showered after dinner, which he prepared. Nevertheless he was happy to have me at home.

Later when the brace was removed a part of his nights was spent massaging my back with liniment when the pain was at its highest level. He became my back, lifting and bending for me, and whenever we went into the car he had to put my left leg in after me. On many occasions he looked at me and said, "Look at the beautiful woman I married, what happened?" I then replied, "When you say for better for worse, you don't expect this kind of worse, do you?"

It seemed inevitable that Charley and I should be married. The first time Charley saw me he told his brother that he had seen his wife. "I have seen my wife tonight" were his exact words. His brother, amazed, asked to whom was he referring. Charley answered, "The same girl that you were dancing with". His brother laughed. I had not seen him that night but had danced with his brother

67

Norris, who told me that he was married with children.

I had arrived in Hartford in December 1971 to live with my mother. The two-family house that we occupied had a very friendly family living downstairs, Mr. and Mrs. Willis with their two daughters Janice and Loretta. Janice introduced me to the *Caribbean Ladies Cultural Club of Hartford*. I fell in love with the club and immediately became a member. The club had many trips and I went on most of them. One remarkable trip was to a place called Peg Leg Bates named after the owner because he had a wooden leg. We boarded the bus that would take us from Hartford to Peg Leg Bates in New York in June 1973.

We dressed in casual clothes for the bus ride there, and then changed into evening dresses when we arrived. To my surprise, the men were admiring me when I walked in dressed in my fancy pink gown sparkling with rhinestones. Charley was in the group with his brother Norris (that was the night I danced with Norris and Charley told him that he had seen his wife), but I did not see him until our return to Hartford. I noticed a man staring straight into my face as he made his exit off the bus, a look I never got from any other man, one that left a lasting impression on my memory. His face was dead serious. As our eyes met, his hazel eyes seemed to penetrate my soul. He did not speak, did not smile only turned and made his exit. He was short, five feet three inches, (too short for me, I had dreamed of marrying a tall man) slim with curly black hair and yellow complexion.

Al was a very good friend of my family, an older man about twenty-five years my senior; we met through my mother because they worked in the same building. He became my dancing partner when I discovered that he was a great dancer. We were not intimate, just good friends who went out for fun. Al and I were at a party out of town on July 21, 1973 seated at a table happily having a drink when the same short yellow complexioned man walked in with some of his friends. They took seats at our table and again he seriously stared dead into my face without speaking or smiling, as he had when he had walked off the bus from Peg Leg Bates. Al and I danced throughout the night, ignoring him. Sometime during the night I noticed he had disappeared. Later he told me that he was upset when he saw me with Al.

December 2, 1973 I attended a dance at the West Indian Social Club on a date with a man whom I later learned was married. There I recognized the short, yellow-skinned man looking at me again for the third time. But this time was different. As soon as my date left the table for the bathroom, he took his seat and asked me for a dance, I declined saying I felt tired. Later, I danced with him. While dancing, he asked for my name and said his name was Charley. I did not like the way he pronounced his name with a Jamaican Patois accent. One of my reasons for leaving Jamaica was to find a foreign husband because I did not want to marry a Jamaican (did not like how some of them treated their wives. They left them at home with the children while they went out partying. Some were also abusive, beating their women. Later, I learned that this happens in all countries). He looks good, I thought to myself but he is too short, still thinking I should marry a tall man. I do not remember what else was said after exchanging our names. When the song ended, I took my seat and he left.

About a week later my friend Al said, "You know who asked me about you, the short man from the club, he wanted to know if I was your boyfriend, should I give him your phone number?" "No, he is too short" I replied. On another occasion, for the second time Al told me the short man asked about me and wanted to get my phone number from him. All forgotten, one night my phone rang it was this man, Charley. I asked where he got my number he said from the telephone directory where there were only two people with the name *Lindo* listed, the first number he dialed was mine. He asked for a date, I declined.

I shared an apartment with my mother and sisters Shirley and Georgia. (Later he told me that my mother had answered the phone that night and asked him if I was expecting his call and he said yes). He was persistent, calling regularly; each time I told him I would not go on a date with him, he would call again. I stopped taking his calls, my sister Shirley begged me to speak to him. "He sounds very lonely," she said. Finally, I decided to go out with him so that he would stop calling. After spending so much time trying to convince me to go out with him, the man showed up late for our first date. We went dancing. When he took me home he asked for another date saying we needed to be even. I really did not want to go on another date with him but found myself out dancing with him for the second time, and then going to the movies for our third date.

On Valentine's Day 1974 he sent me a card that read, "Cupid has our number." At the bottom he wrote,

"Laugh at me Fay." I have to admit that I did. That year I was active in the Methodist church (where my mother and I became members), attending the women's circle meetings, helping with dinners, coffee hour and tag sales, even taking part in a play there, and also being active in the Ladies Cultural Club as a model and the queen. In my first year as a member of the Ladies Cultural Club, the ladies chose me to be the queen to ride on the float in the West Indian Independence parade. Being shy I refused. The following year they choose me again, this time I accepted and represented the club in the parade and at the dance as *Miss Caribbean Ladies Cultural Club 1974.*

Charley told me that he needed to make an appointment to see me because my schedule was always full. I invited him to some of the functions. As I modeled for the Ladies Cultural Club at a church fashion show he could be seen in the audience standing against the wall admiring me. He saw me on the float and told me that I looked beautiful. My float was not as lovely as the float the previous year. It was a sports car decorated with paper and I sat on top of the back seat. Half way on the parade route the car broke down. Another driver who was on his way to the destination of the parade, which was the West

Indian Social Club rescued me.

I could not help reminiscing about the gorgeous float I would have rode on the previous year had I accepted the crown that year. I imagined being seated under the flower-covered arch on the huge float that was beautifully decorated with various flowers wrapped around its body. Now, I sat in a car instead of on a float to complete my journey, hidden from many of my friends and family who were anxiously waiting at the Club to see me wave to them from a pretty float. Some said I should have sat on the hood of the car. However, I arrived at the West Indian Social Club safely, and took my seat on the reviewing stand with the mayor of Hartford and other dignitaries; there I could easily be seen by all the people.

That night Charley accompanied me to the Independence Ball at a classy hotel downtown Hartford where we danced, drank wine, and chattered. And his nightly phone calls continued. His pet name for me was "Lover Doll," he would say, "How are you, Lover Doll?" My mother had returned to Jamaica so he wrote her a letter requesting my hand in marriage as was the custom then. At my then age of twenty-eight and not a virgin I thought that was a respectable thing for him to do.

73

When my mother returned to America, Charley made arrangements to meet her. The night of the meeting, mom and I went to the hospital to visit my sister Georgia who had had knee surgery. We should have left the hospital on time to meet Charley at the house but mom was in no hurry to meet him so, when he went to the house and no one was there, he left his cigarette butt on the step to prove that he had been there. Needless to say that he was very upset that we had stood him up; but he did arrange to meet her another time

Before Charley entered my life there was a man named Roan. He was the first person I met on my arrival in Hartford on December 6, 1971. It was my first morning in town; I was walking down the back stairs with the garbage when I bumped into a short, stout, fairly good-looking man going to visit the landlord. We exchanged hellos as he passed. A few days later someone knocked on my door. To my surprise it was the same man and he introduced himself as Roan. He continued to visit and call asking me for dates until I accepted his invitation to dinner. He told me that he loved me and asked me to marry him many times. His actions showed that he really loved me and my mother liked him but I was not in love with him and thought he was too short so I turned down his marriage proposals. During the following years he visited sometimes, still asking for my hand in marriage. One night I kept a *Mary Kay* party at my apartment and he stopped by to visit. Charley also stopped by at the same time to visit. Both men met face-to-face in my apartment, I had not invited them and had no intention of marrying either one, so I was not worried. Roan said he was not worried because he knew that I would not marry Charley. He left the party before Charley.

I can only say that it was destined for us to be together because I was not madly in love with Charley but somehow I had a feeling that he was to be my husband and I continued to date him as if driven by an unknown force. Soon he introduced me to his big family. His mother had ten children; two died young leaving eight, six boys and two girls. His oldest brother had six children, four girls and two boys, another brother had four boys, another brother had six boys, another had two girls and one boy, one sister had two boys and one girl, and the other sister had two girls. His aunt also had ten children. As time would reveal he was the brother of the man named Norris with whom I had danced at Peg Leg Bates. He lived with

75

Norris and his lovely wife Tamsy and their six children. Tamsy became my good friend and helper. One could never ask for a better person to enter their life. She would not hesitate to take a trip with me on short notice. She helps to clean up at birthday parties and visits anyone who is in the hospital or the convalescent home, always bringing the most beautiful card and a gift. She never misses a birthday or an anniversary. I could expect one of her most magnificent cards with encouraging words on these special occasions.

By October 1974 Charley bought me an engagement ring. His plan was to have a surprise party for my birthday on October 19, and present it to me there, but like a little boy with a new toy he became overly excited and could not keep the secret until then so he showed it to me before. I still remember that night as if it was yesterday; we were in his apartment (he had moved from his brother's house) when he presented what has to be the smallest diamond in the world, and said he told the jeweler to make it smooth that it would not tear my stockings. I said to him, "How can you buy me a ring and you did not ask me to marry you?" He immediately went down on his knees and asked, "Will you marry me?"

The birthday/engagement party took place at his brother's house in October 1974. Our wedding was on February 8, 1975 at the Methodist church where I was a member; the reception was at the now demolished Parkview Hilton Hotel in Hartford, Connecticut. Our honeymoon was in one of the rooms upstairs that night. After the wedding we moved into an apartment building for only one hundred and twenty three dollars per month. Sometime before the wedding a baby had been conceived. One morning I awoke and was overcome by nausea so bad I was about to faint. After rushing to the bathroom and hurriedly washing my face with cold water I was revived. This feeling made me realize that I was pregnant. I felt happy; I love children and wanted four. Charley wanted only one. When I broke the news to him he said he already knew. He seemed to know everything: he knew I was going to be his wife and he knew when I got pregnant.

We decided to get married in the United Methodist church I attended and christen the children in the Catholic Church he attended. My dream of marrying someone from my church did not come true. The United Methodist Women's circle surprised me with a baby shower. My sisters and a friend, Cynthia, threw me a second surprise shower and my department at work gave me a third surprise baby shower. I was blessed with everything that was needed for the baby such as bottles, blankets, bags, clothes, lotions, stroller etc. Charles Jr. arrived in July 1975.

As a young woman, dozens of men were attracted to me. It started in primary school. I remember walking home from school with boys following me like lovesick puppies. When I got older my hobby was counting the number of men who approached me every day, marking the number on the calendar and totaling it at the end of the month. Many had asked for my hand in marriage before I left Jamaica. I wondered if every woman had as many marriage proposals and why so many men wanted to marry me. Later I realized not all women did.

It is said that beauty is in the eyes of the beholder, so I must have been beautiful because everyone who beheld me, both men and women remarked daily how beautiful I was. This must have been the magnet that drew the men to me. With thick black shoulder length hair, some thought that I was an Indian. Many people loved my hair: at school the children were always combing it and adults were always touching it. When Charley and I started dating he would brush it and set it with the rollers whenever he came to visit, then we kissed until they all fell out. He continued to comb it after we were married. Some admired my smile; they said it was beautiful and pleasant. Men often told me that I was "sexy," I did not understand what that meant until someone told me it was because of my big breasts and slim body.

I wonder how many of those men would have coped with my challenges and disability if married to me. Would James, the man who waited seven years for me from I was thirteen until I was twenty have stayed? At that time men asked parents for their daughters. When my mother told him I was only thirteen, he said he would wait for me until I was older. While he waited he visited occasionally informing me that he was dating other women but assured me I was going to be his wife so he would not have sex with them because he was saving himself for me. When I was twenty and still refused to go out with him that was the last he visited. Years after I was married, in telling Charley the story I learned that he and James were good friends. I was about thirty three years old when I saw James again, still not married. He was quite shocked when he heard whom I had married.

79

Taylor

Would Vernon, one of mom's tenants who asked me to marry him when I was about seventeen still be with me, or Kenneth the neighbor who lived across the street and rode his bicycle alongside me in the mornings as I walked to high school handing me love letters that I never took and, being upset he ripped them to pieces?

Lawrence was the assistant scoutmaster from the Methodist Church Boy Scout troop who helped the Girl Guides (called Girl Scouts in America) mistress to teach and test the girls for their badges. I was a member of both the church and the troop. He loved me and waited a few years for a 'yes' to his proposal while he worked with me at Guide meetings, helping me to get my badges and walking me home sometimes after the meetings. As a Girl Guide I learned to be prepared but I was not prepared for the tricks that men played on women. One night he offered to take me home from a party held at the Guide mistress's house. I noticed that the taxi was taking a route that did not lead to my home and asked if he was going to visit someone. I do not remember his answer but recall exiting the taxi with him when it stopped at a house. He told me to wait by the steps while he spoke to a man at the door. What he said next made me realize that this was a hotel. Without hesitation I lied telling him he picked the wrong night to bring me there because I was having my period. He asked if I was serious and I seriously said yes. With much disappointment he took me home.

History repeated itself when the minister who agreed to sign a paper for me said to meet him down town after work. We walked into a place that I had no idea was a hotel, being young and naïve at age twenty-two, a hotel was the farthest thought on my mind. We entered a room where he started to hug and fondle me. I fought him with all my strength. The girdle I was wearing saved me from getting raped as I escaped his hands and nervously bolted out the door. Running to the bus stop I kept looking back to see if he was chasing me. I still remember the floral orange skirt and the black blouse I was wearing that afternoon. My nerves rocked for the remainder of the night. He apologized and said he would still sign the paper. He had a wife and six children. These were secrets I never revealed to anyone.

BD was a singer whom I met at the National Stadium on one of my Girl Guides assignments. He was tall, slim and handsome. He asked me out on a date but I thought singers had many women so I did not go out with

81

him. A friend told me that he asked her about me several times during the following two years. I could not believe he still remembered me.

After leaving Waulgrove College, a high school, I started working at Gem Store as a sales clerk. I had failed my General Certificate of Education (GCE) exam (passing this exam allows one to graduate with a diploma) and not knowing the importance of graduating from high school, decided not to return to take it again, although my mother insisted that I remain in school and repeat the GCE. I had attended for four years and after failing I thought that I was wasting her money (in Jamaica we paid to attend high school). Instead I took a job at a dry goods store working in the lingerie department and attending commercial school at nights doing IBM keypunch, typing, shorthand, and business courses. At the end of the course I graduated with a certificate.

The store became another place for meeting men. Shortly after I started working there, the man who was in charge of the men's department next to the lingerie department started pursuing me. He was tall, good-looking, dark skinned and very chubby. His name was Roan. Whenever sales were slow, he would come over and talk with me. When the fruit vendor stopped in the store he wanted to buy me the best fruits in the basket. He walked with me to the bus stop after work then walked back to his car because I refused to accept his offer to drive me home. His mother owned a lingerie business where she designed and made lingerie then delivered them to the stores. He also helped her with the delivery by bringing them in with him. A part of my job was to receive and check them when they were delivered to Gem Store. This brought us closer and eventually I accepted a ride home in his nice big car with a musical horn. It progressed from rides home after work to rides after school and church. Then he started picking me up at home some mornings to ride with him and his mother to work.

He became my first boyfriend. He spent many nights sitting on the verandah with me just talking. Our nightly drive out took us atop Beverley Hills admiring the bright city lights below, or a trip to the beach where we enjoyed the cool sea breeze, sometimes to a restaurant to get a sandwich. It was about three months before we kissed. He was my first boyfriend but not the first man for me. I did not have the opportunity of losing my virginity to a young man with whom I was in love because an older man had raped me at an early age. Our relationship was already strong when someone told me that he had another woman with two children. When I asked him he admitted it but said they were not together anymore. During the time we were dating I heard that she had given birth to a third child for him. Here began my experiences with romantic pain and how men used women. I asked him why he did not marry her; he said they could not get along. I thought she was stupid to be having all his kids without him marrying her. Lucky for me there were no wedding bells ringing in my head. We remained friends until I left Jamaica. I heard that he married another woman, still did not marry the woman with the kids.

Peter was a short, brown-skinned, half Indian man who came in the store to visit a friend and thought I was an Indian. She told me he was from Chicago. We went on two dates, one to the movies the other to a club. After we left the club he drove to a secluded area, stopped the car and started to undress me. Once again I had to fight since I was not the type to have sex with someone I just met. He asked me to marry him and took me to meet his grandmother with whom he lived. She did not like me and I never went out with him again. Pat, another man who saw me in the store when he stopped in to visit his sister who worked there, also waited three years for an answer. Each time he stopped in to see his sister he would ask me for a date. I finally went to the movies with him once.

Then there was Basil, my favorite. He did the wrapping in the store. He was three years my junior. Tall, slender, very cute, brown complexion, pretty brown eyes, always neatly dressed and had a quiet shy nature. We went to the beach, dancing at a nightclub and we often opened the dance floor at his parties that he had regularly at his house. One day he came to visit me at home and Roan, who I was no longer dating, stopped by to visit. I met Roan at the gate while Basil waited in the house. Later Basil started dating another girl. I left them all and came to America.

When I first came to America I did not meet as many men as in Jamaica. Later, the ones I met were already married. The first one was a rich white man who wanted me to be his mistress. He promised to pay the rent for my apartment, take care of me and my only job was to be there whenever he wanted me. He was astonished when I refused his offer. The second man was Wilson whom I liked a lot, a friend had introduced us. She told me he was not married. After a few dates, one to the Copacabana in New York, one on a boat ride and a dinner date I learned that his wife and kids were in Panama. He was only seeking a visa. Of all the men, Charles Taylor was the one destined to share life's challenges with me, and it's already over thirty years of our struggling together.

I did have some proposals after we were married. Once at a gas station when I stopped to purchase gas the Indian attendant thought I was an Indian judging from the gold bracelets on my hand. He asked nicely if I was married because he was seeking a wife. Another man in the car next to mine at a traffic light questioned if I was married, when I said yes he asked if I needed a lover. The other incident happened on my way to a concert. The policeman who was busy directing traffic stopped to stare at me crossing the street. His eyes followed me across in amazement. Again, at a club a man approached me and asked for my name; when he heard "Taylor" he asked if any relationship to the Taylors I replied, "I am married to Charles." He said o.k.

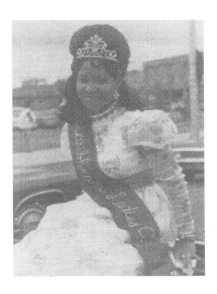

Figure 16: Representing Caribbean Ladies Cultural Club

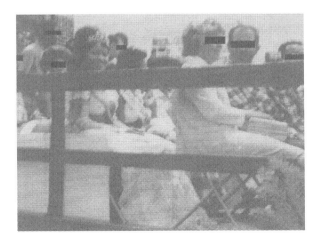

Figure 17: On the reviewing stand with Hartford dignitaries

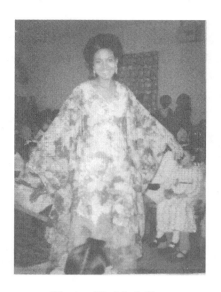

Figure 18: Modeling

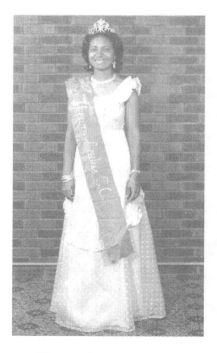

Figure 19: Fay as Queen

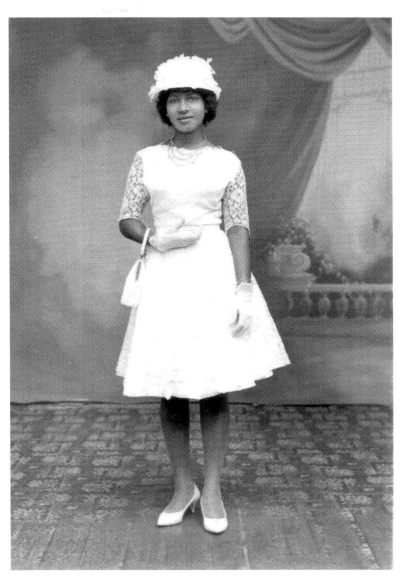

Figure 20: Receiving in church in Jamaica

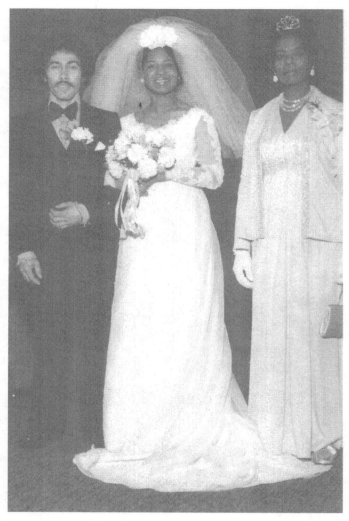

Figure 21: The Wedding

CHAPTER 6

BOWEL, BLADDER AND SEX

W hen the bowel program and the catheterization were being done, I thought they were necessary because of my inability to get out of bed. It never occurred to me that there could be a permanent loss of bowel and bladder function; neither did it occur to the many people who were focused only on my sexual capabilities that my bladder and bowel were dysfunctional. The physiatrist had mentioned a couple of times that my bladder should return to normal when I started walking. This never happened so I continued to cath myself. He said nothing about the bowels, never told me that I would not be able to defecate normally again.

I will always remember that first time; I had just finished lunch, and was alone in my room when I felt the urge to move my bowels. I was filled with surprise at having actually felt this; I asked the nurse if I should wait for the bowel program or should I use the toilet. (As I mentioned before, every night they did a bowel regime by inserting a suppository then manually removing the waste). She too, was surprised that I had the urge and said that was good; by all means use the toilet. But only the feeling was there; I could not go. That's when my potty training began. She brought in the plastic gloves and surgical lubricant and taught me how to disimpact myself. The same procedure the nurses had been doing nightly in the bowel program, I would have to do for the rest of my life. This was the hardest thing to accomplish especially with the body jacket still on; I had to put extra stretch on my arm. During this period I discovered that I had no sensation in my rectum. The hemorrhoids that popped out were painless; I had no knowledge of them until the nurse mentioned that I needed medication to treat them.

Catheterization was a more complicated and awkward process. I had to raise the head of the bed, lean against pillows, set up the kit, and place a mirror between my legs to see the urethra so that I could insert the tube called "catheter." Using rubber gloves, I cleaned around the urethra five times with soft cloths dipped in povidone-iodine solution before inserting the catheter. After catherization, the area had to be cleaned once again. Since I was concerned about doing this at home, my nurse suggested that I talk to another accident victim who had the same problem.

She was a beautiful woman who was involved in a car accident with her family. Her husband and children were fine, but she was paralyzed. She assured me not to worry, that it was easy; she could now cath by feeling. Was that possible? I could not imagine how that could be done. Later the nurse taught me the "Clean Cath Method," in which the kit and gloves were eliminated and I used my bare hands that were washed clean to do the catheterization. Long after being at home, my medical doctor, Dr. McCoy suggested that I learn to catheterize by feeling. I told him that was impossible. One of the lessons I learned from this accident is to try to do things that have been suggested. I took his advice and tried. It worked; I graduated from sitting on the bed with a mirror between my legs, to being an expert, cathing on the toilet. Whenever I take a trip somewhere, and have to urinate, I give credit to Dr. McCoy as I go in search of a bathroom and not a bed.

Having to catheterize myself every two to three hours and never being able to empty my bowels completely annoy me sometimes. It seems like most of my time is being spent in the bathroom. The terrible headaches and backaches that accompany the problems in moving my bowel is a personal misery no one would understand. There is also the financial burden, which comes with this package. As the years go by, my expenses for the medical supplies escalate. The list includes rubber gloves, surgical lubricant, sponges, iodine prep solution, *Hibiclens®* soap, hemorrhoidal pads, adult undergarment, and catheters. These items have become as necessary to me as food is necessary for my body. Life could be miserable if I allowed it to be. Instead, I fight the feeling of self-pity and move on. It was months after I was home that my sister Georgia told me that the doctor in Philadelphia told her I would not have bladder and bowel functions, yet no one had told me this when I was in the hospital. Eventually, I had surgery to correct the incontinence, but I still use a catheter.

Many people were curious about my sex life, whether it was possible to have sex with a Spinal Cord Injury and a broken back. However, none was as explicit as my neighbor Theresa. When she visited me, she immediately blurted the words, "Can you have sex?" I had not imagined this being a problem until she asked the question.

Charley and I were good sex partners; we made love often. As I mentioned, we had done it three times between the time we arrived at the resort and the following morning. We had planned to continue this trend for the weekend. Unfortunately, those three times were the last of my sexual experience as the accident caused a loss of sensation in my vaginal area. Approximately eight months after the accident, still wearing my body jacket, we tried to make love, Charley said, "I can't do this, I feel like I am having sex with a robot." On the second try, he exclaimed, "I can't do this, I feel like I am having sex with a dead person." It took many trial periods before we became comfortable with the situation, and he has coped very well with the problems during intercourse. The sessions at the Spinal Cord Injury (S.C.I) meetings about sex did not interest him. He was not about to try anything new. Several things were suggested but one thing I remember was putting some whip cream in the navel which sounded like pornography to him, so he forbids me to attend another meeting. In answer to the question that many people ask, "Can you have sex," the answer is yes, my sex life has resumed, but it's different with the spinal cord injury. It is not as enjoyable and we seldom do it because of my back pain.

CHAPTER 7

EMBARASSING MOMENTS

W hen a friend of mine visited me in the rehab hospital, he listened attentively while I explained how the accident happened. I was describing how my back hit the rock when suddenly his back hit the floor. He had fainted; the nurses rushed in and revived him. I heard the hospital sent him a bill.

We have all experienced embarrassing moments in our lives. Some we can bypass; other times we wished that the earth would open so that we could disappear. I have accepted some of the most embarrassing moments with a smile, because of the accident. Although I was in pain, I still had my pride, so when a young white male nurse started to wash my private area, naturally, I objected. I wanted a female nurse to do it because that's what I was accustomed to. However, he insisted that there was no other nurse available, and that was the first of many embarrassing moments. My second encounter was when the men were putting on and trimming the cast. Having to lie there exposed and helpless to many different men was no fun.

The bowel and bladder dysfunction contributed to most of my embarrassment. As I mentioned before, I was not aware of the problems in this area; therefore I did not know that they would move without my control. One day my therapist, Deena, was going to do therapy with me, I had just finished the board transfer from the wheelchair to the mat on which she was about to do my therapy, when she noticed that feces had been in the wheelchair, on the board and on the mat. Another therapist immediately picked up the board and Deena said, "Do not use that board." With a smile he started off with it and she said, "I am serious, do not use it." She then put a red marker on the mat to inform the other therapists that it had to be cleaned before they could use it for their patients. There are no adjectives to describe how I felt. The other incident that involves the bowel is the night I had diarrhea. As fast as the female nurse changed the sheets and washed me I would be dirty again. She became upset at my continuous request for her help and refusal of the male nurse, and told me it was his job as well as hers, and she would not be doing it alone all night.

Taylor

One day I proudly stepped down the hall in Gaylord as I did my daily walk, not realizing that the large adult pad I wore due to my incontinence was bulging. "Fay, I did not know that you had changed your sex," exclaimed one of the nurses. Changed my sex, what is she talking about?" I wondered. "You are well endowed, you are the man I would like to have," she continued. Looking down, I saw the bulge that was made by the undergarment and realizing what she meant used a smile to cover my embarrassment, because it was meant to be funny.

On many occasions I have had to change clothes due to my incontinence. My first experience with this was at a function in a club, as I stood up, the urine made its way down my legs to the floor. This was when I realized that I had to travel with a change of clothing. Luckily my sister, who was with me, had an extra pair of pants in her car that matched perfectly with the top I was wearing. On another occasion my husband and I drove to New York to visit family I had never met. Overjoyed to see us they greeted us by the car when we arrived. We were hugging and kissing each other when suddenly I felt the urine flowing down. Excusing myself I left the gathering and rushed to the bathroom to change. Also at a family picnic I had left my seat to go inside the house when someone told me that the back of my pants was soaked. Due to the lack of sensation in my rear I have no knowledge of what goes on in that area and after sitting for a long period of time, my bladder runs like an open faucet.

There is also the inability to control my flatus, which chooses to expel in public at all times. Usually in quiet places, like in the church at my sister's wedding and in the attorney's office at the refinancing of our home.

Although I had grown accustomed to it, I was never comfortable with the different nurses washing and catheterizing me. Having to lie helpless, as the many different people handled my body was very embarrassing.

FEARS

I didn't have many fears. Only three specific ones stand out in my mind, two of which I mentioned earlier: fear of the Heparin injections below my navel, and fear of caring for myself at home. The third was not being able to run if there was a fire. Ironically, the alarm went off one night as the nurse started to catheterize me (empty my bladder). She ran off leaving the catheter inside my urethra. When she returned she said another nurse told her she had run off leaving a spoon in a patient's mouth, and she answered, "Really? I left a tube sticking into Fay." Although I was shaken I managed to laugh.

Sometimes patients in wheelchairs were taken on trips outside of the hospital and offered an ice cream treat. On one of those trips, the driver had loaded the van, strapped in the wheelchairs, closed the door and was about to drive, when one girl blurted out, "I do not want to go!" The driver, now tired from loading, asked if she was serious, and she replied, "Yes." He told her he would drive around the hospital grounds first; then if she did not change her mind he would not take her. Driving around the hospital grounds did not help, because she had been in a car accident and as she sat in the van she had flashbacks. On this windy day it was no fun for him to remove her and reload the van, because she was in the front. I felt compassion for her; how would she travel again I thought, this was a fear I prayed she would overcome. In the same way that she was afraid to ride in a car, I am afraid to ride a horse again.

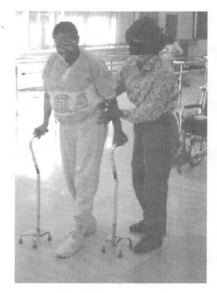

Figure 22: Therapy with Deena

CHAPTER 8

LESSONS LEARNED

I t is my understanding that there are lessons to be learned from our calamities. One important lesson I learned was that simple every day tasks we take for granted in our lives while we are healthy become impossible to accomplish when we are disabled. This I learned the day my left leg slipped off the bed and I was unable to lift it regardless of my efforts. Having to call someone to replace it, I found myself laughing although it was not funny.

Another lesson is that the closeness of family relationship is essential. We cannot function alone, we need each other. I would not have made it through those tough times without my family, their love, support, visits, gifts and encouraging words. The other fact is to never give up, keep trying. Had I not tried, many things that I can do now would have to wait until someone could do it for me. Like doing the laundry, driving a car and cooking a meal.

The adage, "If life gives you lemons, make lemonade" proved true with me. Focusing on the good that resulted from the accident instead of the bad has helped me to move smoothly through life. It's not an experience I wanted to have, nor would wish on my enemy, but since it has happened, I have accepted it and have never looked back for long. Whenever wandering thoughts enter my mind such as, "Wonder what life would have been like if I did not have the accident," I quickly replace them with the thoughts, "It's already happened, move on." My temporary confinement to a wheelchair allows me to understand how the people who must occupy one permanently feel. Having to live with an injured spinal cord gives me the knowledge of what others with this injury experience.

An accident as life altering as mine reminds me of how my view of the world has changed, how humble I feel as I make my way through an ordinary day. A trip to the supermarket, the mall or perhaps a restaurant becomes easier for me when I legally park in a "Handicap Access" spot, thus giving me easy access to places I need to go. I admit that I had grouched and grumbled about these "reserved" parking places, especially when they were empty and I was in a hurry. I confess! I am embarrassed to admit my insensitivity to those faceless people who need these special places. When I joined the ranks of the permanently disabled, my attitude changed. I understand on a much deeper level that I am fortunate enough to be able to drive and that others are worse than I am. My accident taught me to be thankful for what I have and never criticize the world for a small inconvenience that could come back to haunt me.

In the midst of my problems the strength and courage that helped me heal came from my awareness of my blessings. In a conversation with a friend months after I was home, she said it surprised her when she asked, "Why you, Fay?" that I remarked, "Why not me?" Accidents happen every day, why not me?

I won't ever forget July 29, 1989. The scars remain visible and I will continue to live with the permanent damage from my accident forever. But I have learned that love, support and hard work define the quality of life. If this is "Luck" I have plenty of it. One nurse had told me that I was the first person with a spinal cord injury of that magnitude to walk out of Gaylord Hospital. That is a miracle.

CHAPTER 9

BROKEN TWICE

I t is the opinion of many people that I became a millionaire from this accident because the place where we stayed in the Poconos is a big resort. They thought I sued and won millions of dollars. I wish this were so.

While at Gaylord Hospital I hired a local attorney in Connecticut who then recommended me to (in his opinion) one of the best attorneys in Pennsylvania (in my opinion he was one of the worst).

According to my new attorney the stables were owned by a private person and had a different name from the resort. Although horseback riding was printed on their brochure as one of the activities available to their customers they were not affiliated with the stables. He said that the Pocono resort could not be sued because of a certain clause that prevented such a suit. According to Pennsylvania law, businesses could obtain certain waivers which would prevent them being sued. I could sue the stables but they were not responsible for my damages since it could not be proven that it was their fault. The first reason they threw at me was that I had signed a waiver releasing the stable from any liability. I did not sign any papers but Charley did sign one, which they said represented the both of us. We managed to pass that hurdle and after writing a statement about what exactly happened, at their request, they sent me some interrogatories that I completed while in extreme pain. The next step was the pre-trial which I could not attend since it was held in Pennsylvania. My attorney informed me by telephone that they made an offer, which I refused and told him I would rather go to trial, he exclaimed, "You want more?"

At times I wondered if he had my best interest at heart or the stable's. Reason being, he did not send me statements from witnesses (which I requested) until the case was closed. Also such remark as it was a poor stable and was insured for only three hundred thousand dollars (later I learned that it was three hundred thousand dollars per person), which I could not get due to other law suits against them, led me to this decision. Two years later the stables filed for bankruptcy, leaving me with about thirty

Taylor

thousand dollars in doctor and hospital bills after my health insurance paid.

The bankruptcy suit did not stop a deposition. Since I wasn't able to travel to Pennsylvania, the attorneys traveled to Hartford, Connecticut to the office of my local attorney. This was close to my home. The day the deposition was taken, my pain was at its highest level. Unable to sit, I used the couch in the office as a bed while awaiting their arrival. During the deposition there was no comfortable position for me. I moved around like an overactive little girl; sliding down in a lying position, sitting up straight, turning sideways, standing behind the chair, sitting again, standing against the wall then sitting again. This behavior continued throughout the questioning and at one point one of the attorneys said, "I notice you are moving around, is it because you are in pain?" My attorney had told me before the deposition started that I could stop when I wasn't feeling well. Since I was always in pain I figured there wasn't a right time for this, so I just suffered through it to the end.

Being the only woman among all men (the reporter taking the notes, the attorney representing the Pocono resort, the attorney for the stables, my attorney and my husband) and being in extreme pain, it was not easy to cope with all the questions they asked. Questions too numerous to list, my life story starting from my birth, my family's life story starting from their birth, their health record, my relatives' life story starting from birth, their health record and educational background. Questions that I thought were not relevant to the accident, like where did I meet my husband, did I gain weight because of my inactivity and did I return home to Jamaica for my Green Card. Every large and minute question about the accident was not missed. The most private question was how often I had sex before the accident and the number of times per week I had sex since the accident. The most insulting question was, did I know that the horse was an animal. The most ridiculous was, which hand was in front of the other when I held the rein; was the right in front of the left or vice versa. In all fairness, was I suppose to remember that?

Later my attorney informed me that they upped the offer a little more and his advice would be to take it and run because they had filed for bankruptcy and it wasn't a good idea to go to court. He said if I went to court there was a possibility of losing it all since the jury would be awarding money that the stables did not have. Charley sued for being without the society and companionship of his wife and was not even considered in the suit. The small settlement was meant for the both of us. After lawyer fees and the other expenses were paid, I was left practically broke.

I had survived the tragedy and with a smile accepted the award life had handed me. I did not lose my faith; my quest would be to discover the reason. There wasn't time for my discovery because the problems kept gushing into my life like water from a broken pipe. Why was I faced with all these challenges? Was I supposed to be the next Job? (A man mentioned in the Bible who had endurance to resist temptation) I wondered.

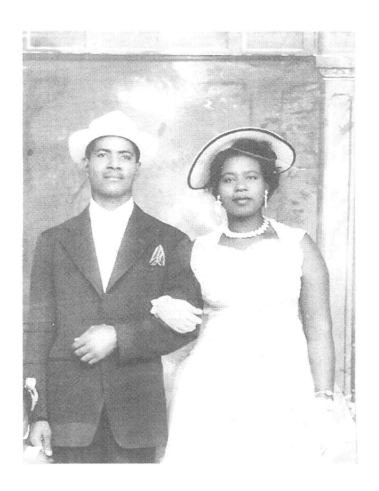

Figure 23: A.R. and Urceline Lindo

CHAPTER 10

MY FATHER

I t was only one year and eleven days since my accident. I was still going to different doctors for follow up visits. On August 9, 1990 my sister Georgia and I had stopped to visit our mother on our way home from Yale New Haven Hospital where I had just completed my bladder study. We were shocked when mom said, "Your father was hit by a car while riding his bicycle and he is in the hospital." "How bad is he?" I asked. "His neck is broken," came her reply.

He was in the intensive care unit when we arrived at a local hospital in Hartford. We could not see him and when we were allowed in, only one person at a time could go in. My mother, four sisters, two brothers and I kept vigil at the hospital for hours. His condition was extremely critical. Diagnosis was: broken neck, broken nose, one leg broken in three places, left ear badly damaged, later we learned, fractured back and brain injury.

112

As I looked down at my father in extreme pain, memories of my accident became vivid. The words "I know exactly how you feel" came from my mouth, while simultaneously realizing how he must have felt when he stood on the other side of the bed looking down at me and he said, "I can't bear to see you like that."

While he was in the intensive care unit the cervical traction they had put on his head to stabilize his neck was too high and had to be replaced by another. This made two new holes; he then went to surgery where a halo was put on. That halo was removed because it could not go into the MRI scanner. A new halo was put on allowing him to go into the scanner. This made four more holes, making a total of twelve holes in his head.

It was approximately three weeks before he was removed from the intensive care unit to a regular room. He was in the local hospital for approximately two months, with new complications arising daily; on Monday August 13, 1990, he had heart failure, low oxygen level and low blood pressure. Tuesday the 14th, the back fracture and internal bleeding were discovered. Thursday the 16th, the halo was taken off to do the brain scan. The results showed Hematoma on the brain. This meant another surgery to remove the blood. After this surgery he went into a coma for about two weeks. When he awoke, his memory was lost. He did not recognize any of us. He didn't know where he was or what had happened to him. At this point he was diagnosed with brain injury.

In my opinion it was during the insertion of the traction that his brain got injured, not from the accident. I strongly believe this because when I saw him in the intensive care unit on the night of the accident, he had explained how the accident happened. He said the man had run the red light while he was crossing. He had been baking buns and was going to the store to get one more ingredient that he needed. He never made it to the store. He also asked me to check on the mixture he had left on the kitchen counter. After the surgery he knew nothing and was diagnosed with brain injury.

Other complications that occurred during this period were; seizures, low heart rate, fluid around the lungs and pneumonia. Never knowing what the next diagnosis would be or what to expect on a visit became nerve racking for the family.

Having to deal with a brain-injured person was new to me so I was not prepared for what happened when I went to visit the man I knew as my father. He looked me straight in the face and asked me, "Do you work here?" Not only was I shocked, but also hurt. This was the day I decided that my visits were a waste of time and I would not go back to visit until he knew who was standing at the side of his bed. "That's not how it works," said my sister Georgia, "You must keep up with the visits. We all must visit daily and talk to him in order to motivate him." She was right. He eventually recognized us. However, sometimes he misplaced our names with our faces. He called Shirley, Georgia. He called LaVerne, Babylin and our mother Urceline, he thought she was our aunt, Cysylin.

Shortly after he awoke from his coma, he told us about his dream. He dreamt that he was locked into a box about to be buried, but he kicked the box open yelling, "It's not time for me to die." At first there were monsters around the box, but later there came angels, and he sang a religious song. While explaining, he started singing the song in a loud voice. We were stunned that he remembered that song so well. We interpret the dream to mean that he had a near death experience, and was given another chance in life.

On one of our visits, Georgia noticed an infection in two of the holes in the front of his head. She pointed this out to one of the nurses who thought it was fine, nothing to worry about. A few weeks later he was transferred to Gaylord Rehabilitation Hospital in Wallingford, the same hospital where I had spent three months the previous year. I had been there before as a visitor, visiting my co-worker Sly, then as a patient, once again I became a visitor.

On dad's second day at Gaylord he became unresponsive because of the infection in his head, and his blood, as well as a urinary tract infection and had to be rushed to MW Hospital. There he remained unresponsive for four days. A doctor asked us to sign a DNR (do not resuscitate) paper in case his heart failed they would not try to save his life because he was brain dead. We refused to do so. The doctor discontinued everything stating that he was the doctor. We dismissed him. The new doctor started antibiotic for his Sepsis. Within two days of the new antibiotics the infection cleared.

The rain was pouring outside when we visited one morning; the man who I thought was not going to regain consciousness was sitting up in the bed looking out of the window. As we walked in he calmly said, "It is raining."

Once again his memory was back. Needless to say how surprised we were to see him sitting up and talking.

After approximately two weeks in MW Hospital he was transferred back to Gaylord Rehabilitation Hospital where he walked after about two months of intensive therapy. Thank God he walked again; this would have been a perfect life for us all if the seizures did not continue. These seizures were scary. He did not fall and shake or foam at the mouth. He would fall and lay stiff with his eyes rolled back as if he was dead. They lasted a few minutes before he returned to normal not knowing what had happened.

Finally it was time for him to be discharged from Gaylord Hospital. We were faced with the challenge of caring for him since he could not be left alone because the seizures would not cease. Mom had not been living with him for many years, they were separated and she was working. My sisters and brothers all worked. The only person not working was me and that was because of my injury. It was impossible for me to assume the responsibility of caring for him at home. Although we all hated to put him in a convalescent home, that was my decision. They all rebelled, especially my brother Hugh.

The thought of seeing his dad in a convalescent home almost destroyed him. Someone suggested we hire a companion helper to live in, care for him and do his housekeeping. Hence a new problem was born. Due to their demand for high salary, special food and certain days off it became a chore finding someone. My sister Georgia and I interviewed many women. Whenever we thought that this matter was settled, the person hired would quit and we had to start over again.

He was not happy with this arrangement; he felt he was healthy enough to live by himself and could return to his usual lifestyle. This included returning to work and riding his bicycle. He complained about the presence of the helpers and the money being paid to them. He questioned whose money was being used to pay them. When he learned that the money was from his savings, he said it was a waste of money because he was capable of caring for himself.

He continued to improve, even cooked meals for himself and the helpers, took his medications independently, traveled to Jamaica with the family and released me as his conservator. The judge at the probate court admiring his strength and his will to be independent, happily granted his wish. One and a half year later, a nurse from the local community homemaker program advised us to stop the companion helper, allow him to live alone, and attend adult day care with supervision in the mornings and evenings. An aide would dress him in the mornings; put him on the senior van for the daycare then return to oversee him in the evenings. My job was to keep his medication box filled daily. He took *Phenobarbital* and *Tegretol* for the seizures, *Motrin* for the arthritis, *Digoxin* for his heart, *Lasex* for water retention and *Colace*, a stool softener.

This plan worked fine for a while, until he opened his door to a woman who he thought he knew. In a struggle to rob him, she pushed him down causing him to break his ninth rib. This was the beginning of his deterioration. We were back where we started, interviewing companion helpers and taking him to different doctors again. We encountered lots of problems with him. He was cutting and burning himself. He passed out and could not open the door for the homemaker to enter. At this point he was hospitalized so that they could evaluate his passing out and the burns on his hands and face. We discovered he got the burns when he passed out while cooking, only to wake up to find the food on the stove on fire. He tried to put it out but only succeeded in burning himself. He was then transferred from the hospital to the nursing home which he had been on the waiting list for.

My father had retired twice and still held a job at the age of seventy-five. He rode a bicycle to and from work in any weather; rain, sun or snow. He also used his bicycle to go grocery shopping and visit friends and family. Not worrying about the distance, he rode miles from Hartford to Windsor and Bloomfield. In the little box tied to the back of his bicycle were cakes and buns that he baked and was happy to deliver. Unfortunately, it was that same bicycle that caused his life to be ruined.

As a seaman, he had survived a storm at sea. He also had survived being run over by a car as he crossed the road. However, when he was hit while riding his bicycle, no one expected him to live. Witnesses reported that on impact he was thrown as high as the traffic light then landed on the hood of the car that struck him and finally he landed on the pavement. He was only one block from his apartment when it happened.

Dad's illness became a strain, stress and pressure on all of us, but mostly me. Not only because I am the eldest of the seven children, but because I was the closest to him and knew more about his business than the others. When it was time to choose a conservator, the family made the unanimous decision that I should be his conservator. This position served as another lesson in my life.

I learned the responsibilities of a conservator, which includes bookkeeping, spending someone else's money, reporting to lawyers, dealing with the state department, probate court, convalescent homes, making pre-funeral arrangements, and hiring home care help. Many sleepless nights were spent writing letters and recording how his money was used, the bills I paid and the things I bought for him. During the days, many hours were spent on the phone making arrangements and appointments with doctors, lawyers, social workers and informing family members about what I was doing.

Within a short time many people had entered his life: Nurses, doctors, therapists, meals on wheels, home health aides, homemakers, lawyers and a judge. Within three years he had been in four different hospitals, twice in one (for his broken neck and cataract surgery), twice in another (for prostate surgery and breast surgery. Lumps had developed in his breasts from one of the medications),

121

a rehabilitation hospital, a day care and two convalescent homes.

We transferred him from Kings Convalescent Home to Holiday Home and Hospital because we wanted the best care for him. There I attended meetings and visited regularly, often bringing him home cooked meals and fresh carrot juice, which he used to make daily.

In spite of all his complications he remained as strong as an ox. On many visits the nurses told me of his strength. Sometimes it took three people to attend to him. On one occasion he was found in the bed with the wheelchair on his back still strapped on because he could not loosen the restraint. My sister Georgia spoke of him as the cat with nine lives, my husband called him the coyote in "The Road Runner." I referred to him as a yo-yo. Mother remarked in a conversation, "Now that he has become a permanent fixture." Four months had passed, his strength decreased from sitting in the convalescent home yet once when I brought him to my house for a home visit he was able to help me cream the butter and sugar with a wooden spoon, no mixer, when I baked a cake. Before the woman pushed him down, he had walked stronger than me because I needed my cane. He always remarked on my cane, "I hate to see you with that stick. When are you going to stop using it?" He said.

His being in the convalescent home did not stop us from involving him in the family gatherings and parties. He attended my husband's 50th birthday party, my mother's birthday party, had Christmas and Thanksgiving dinners at home, celebrated his 80th birthday with a family party at home and attended his youngest son, Hugh's wedding. We all prayed that he would live to attend this wedding, because his health was fluctuating like the stock market. On many occasions we thought he would not be alive the next minute. At the wedding, we gathered to take a family picture. Before the camera went off Papa passed out on the floor. This caused a commotion. Strangers probably thought he had died, but we knew that it was a seizure. It took only a few minutes for him to take part in the festivities again.

While my father sat in the convalescent home, restrained to prevent falling, my heart hurt when I visited him and my mind was troubled when I didn't. I really did not want to visit him because I could not bear to see him withering slowly. Existing but not living, being alive but not able to move around. Being treated like a child as they fed him, changed his diapers and changed his clothes. Yet I continued to visit, although many times he did not recognize me. I had feelings of guilt when I didn't visit him. On one of my visits he begged the nurse to take him to the bathroom but she made him wait for over an hour as the nurses changed shifts. When I mentioned to an aide how long he had been waiting, she told me that he had to wait and that he had on a diaper so he could go in it. Eventually he started urinating into his diaper, and then he was made to sit in it for hours before it was changed. At times he had such bad odor it made me sick. This led to skin breakdown. After a meal his hands, face and the table from which he ate were not cleaned. Sometimes it took me a few minutes to remove the foods that were dried on. My complaints fell on deaf ears.

The trips to visit him, caring for him and the return trips were mild compared to my feelings as I watched this strong man deteriorate. My suffering was more than his since he was not aware of his condition and was free of pain.

When I called my friends to inform them of my father's death, I tried hard not to use the word "finally" because each time we thought he had expired (at least four times), he bounced back stronger as if he had taken a deep sleep and rejuvenated. It has been said to let go of children when they are grown, some still find it hard to do so, now we must learn to let go of our older parents when it is time for them to go. I preferred to see my father die than to sit in the convalescent home in that condition. For this reason I felt some relief when A. R. Lindo passed through death into life eternal on September 27, 1997 at the age of 82.

One request that my father had that I regret not being able to fill was for him to see Jamaica once again as he usually visited every year.

MY MOTHER

My mother was the proudest woman I ever knew. Certain people she did not speak to and told us not to "mix" with them as if we were of a better stock. She always dressed like a queen, seldom wearing the same outfit twice. As a dressmaker she made a dress in one night and had it ready to wear the next day. She also made matching hats with some of the outfits. I truly believe that she had been a queen in another life. She was very sophisticated with a certain class that was different from most people, wanting only the finest things that life offered. She was also a private person who did not want anyone to see her naked.

My mother got married at the tender age of sixteen to a man fifteen years older because she wanted freedom from her parents. When my father asked for her hand in marriage, she thought she would be free to go out and have fun, to do what she desired without restriction. Instead she became pregnant with me and had a more restrained life. She went on to have six more children, making a total of seven, five girls and two boys. She told them to show me respect and call me "Sister Fay" because I was the oldest. Soon everyone was calling me Sister Fay. She called me "Fayco" and dad called me "Fay Fay."

Mom saved for and bought our first home where she opened a dry goods store in the front room. It was stacked with fabric, dresses she made, and a variety of other sewing accessories like threads and zippers. It was at this house that I learned to save at the "Penny Bank" for children in the school not far from where we lived. Every Monday evening after school I stood in line to deposit my small change in my little bankbook.

Shortly after, she sold that house and bought another house with a storefront in which she continued with her dry goods store, by then I was old enough to assist her after school. I liked selling in the store, measuring fabric and helping customers. Several important events, which took place at this home on Pretoria Road, stand out in my mind. That's where my period started and mother told me, "Don't let any boys touch you now." Our neighbor James asked mom for my hand in marriage at the age of thirteen; He knew I was too young but he was willing to wait until I was matured. Mom sent me a birthday greeting on the radio for my sixteenth birthday, my first big birthday party celebration and my first kiss.

Mother's motto of "Good better best, never let it rest until your good is better and your better is best," led her to sell the house on Pretoria Road and purchase a bigger one with a bigger shop on the property. She opened a grocery store, hired someone to help her in it and hired a helper for the housework. She rented three rooms to strangers and occupied four rooms. We had lovely living and dining rooms, two bedrooms, two bathrooms, a front verandah, and a large kitchen. Mom decided to let the tenants use the kitchen. She transformed an area next to the dining room into a kitchen for our use. There were lots of fruit trees throughout the yard: mangoes, tamarind, guinnep, soursop, ackee and breadfruit. The front was decorated with flowers and two large evergreen trees that we decorated at Christmas. In the back we had chicken coops filled with chickens. We always had fresh eggs and chicken to eat.

When television came to Jamaica my mother was the first person in the neighborhood to own one. On Friday nights the neighborhood children flocked to our house to watch *Dr. Kildare* and *Bonanza*. As if at a movie theatre, the living room door was opened to accommodate the crowd that took their seats on the verandah. Those were fun times that we anticipated every weekend.

She was a very strict mother who encouraged us to get an education before getting a companion and paid for us to attend high school. We were not allowed to date at an early age or to go out partying. However, she brought some fun to us by taking us on trips to Hope Gardens, a beautiful botanical garden with hundreds of trees and flowers. After touring the grounds, finding our way through the maze, and viewing the different species of birds we picnicked on the grass. She also had "Outings" when she rented a truck and took a group from Kingston to other parishes. These trips served as both business and pleasure. The beers and sodas were sold and there was a cost to go on the trip. We had fun driving in the back of the truck sitting on make shift seats, singing, joking and drinking sodas and beer. At the destination, usually a beach, we ate rice and peas and chicken or curried goat and rice after a swim in the sea. Sometimes we went to a beach where we could also dance and then a tired but fun filled group returned to Kingston. Another great time I thoroughly enjoyed was going to the triple bill movies on Tuesday nights at the Ritz Theatre. After the movies we walked home in groups chattering and laughing.

I got a chance to go out more than my siblings when I joined the Girl Guides (called Girl Scouts in America). As a member of the Methodist Church I joined the church troop. The idea of joining came to me when the Queen of England visited Jamaica. The girls dressed in blue uniforms formed a fence to keep the crowd from the motorcade and had full view while I was fighting the crowd to see. One of the best decisions I ever made was to become a Girl Guide. It allowed me some freedom and added adventure to my life. Camping, attending many functions, some at the National Stadium and at King's House, which is the Governor General's home, meeting new people and learning new things to achieve badges. I was promoted to patrol leader and was proud to carry the flag on special occasions such as when we marched in parades.

Guides were also required to wear uniforms and march into church every third Sunday, the color party leading with the flags. After the meetings on Thursdays we walked home in groups singing and having fun as we walked. One of the girls in the group was my best friend Lorna whom I met in primary school and have remained friends with over the years until today. Another girl was named Rita; later she introduced me to her boyfriend Robert and said they were traveling as performers. He turned out to be the great Reggae artist Bob Marley; she married him and became the famous Rita Marley. When she introduced him to me that day in Gem Store where I was working, he did not have the dreadlocks.

I was fortunate to attend the Girl Guides Golden Jubilee in 1965, celebrating the 50th Anniversary of guiding in Jamaica. Guides came from many countries including the United States of America, England and Canada to celebrate this special occasion with us. For two weeks we camped at Polo Grounds at Up Park Camp and participated in lots of activities, which the news media followed. The Guide leaders gave us souvenirs to mark the occasion. I still have my gold colored pen with the date inscribed on it. We also exchanged souvenirs like badges and pins with the girls who were visiting. Some of the best times of my life were as a Girl Guide.

My father continued to travel, returning home occasionally bringing us everything to make life more comfortable. Added to the American dollars he brought, he also brought a refrigerator, clothes, food items and souvenirs such as wooden sculptures and ashtrays from different countries. When dad returned home from a long trip overseas it was like Santa Claus arriving at Christmas. We were all excited and gathered to see what he brought. Still lingering in my memory are the tours he gave us on the big ships. They were so fascinating I asked him to get me a job on the ship when I left school. He said that was not a place for a young woman to work. But the seed was already planted; someday I would take a cruise on one of those big beautiful ships and see the world just like my father. This dream was materialized many years later when I was able to take my first cruise to some of the Caribbean Islands.

On one of dad's trips home he opened a small restaurant downtown specializing in fresh fruit juices. He hired people to work there and asked mom to oversee it. He also bought a car for his transportation whenever he was home. The grocery store was closed due to poor choice of management. The people there still owe us money for goods charged to their account. The shop was then divided into two parts, another dry goods store and a bar. Someone was hired to sell in the bar and mom cared for the store while overseeing dad's little restaurant. I helped in the store after school but did not like going into the bar, especially because of the advances from the men.

My parents had three businesses opened at the same time and dad was still working on the ship. With dad away, mom was both mother and father to the seven children while overseeing the businesses. It is no wonder that her nerves failed at one point causing her to hit me with a plate. I saw the plate approaching my face and lifted my hand to guard my face. The plate then broke on my hand making an open wound that sent me to the emergency room. Some nerves were damaged; I got seven stitches and a sling to wear for about two weeks. I was not aware that she could get arrested for it until I was told by family members to tell the doctors another story. I told the doctor my hand went through a window, he laughed. I was a teenager in high school and was teased by my peers who asked if my injury was from my boyfriend's beating. Mom felt badly about it and preferred that I do not talk about the incident. This made my third scar.

The bar soon became enticing to thieves and actually every night they broke in and emptied its contents. When an alarm was installed, they cut the wires during the day and entered in the night. Mom had a telephone in the house and was able to call the police. So often did they break in that mother knew many of the police just by reporting the theft. This was one of her reasons for leaving Jamaica along with the thought that life could be better for her and her children in America.

She came to America to work with a family who sponsored her. I came shortly after to another family who sponsored me. My brothers and sisters were left in the care of our grandaunt until mom was able to have them

Taylor

join her in America. She worked two jobs, saved and sent for my brothers, sisters and my father. Finally the family was together again. She became an evangelist, preached in a small church and ministered to people in the local nursing homes.

Many years later mom was diagnosed with Sarcoidosis, that is, an autoimmune disease that can affect the lung causing her difficulty breathing. She accepted and tried to live with this condition the best way she could. While she continued to work she developed a back problem. She had been postponing her back surgery because of fear due to the Sarcoidosis. While contemplating back surgery she was diagnosed with Ovarian Cancer. She had observed the spotting and thought she was too old to have a period. She was operated on immediately. The doctor told her he had removed all of the cancer.

After a short recovery, the back surgery was performed making it two surgeries in the same year. The first surgery was on March 7, 1995, the second on November 7, 1995. Two years later on June 28, 1997 she was admitted for an intestinal blockage. She went home on July 4, 1997 and was admitted again on July 6, 1997.

134

She had not recovered from either the back problem or the Sarcoidosis when she developed steroid induced diabetes, hypertension, osteoporosis, osteoarthritis, and cardiomyapathy from the steroid taken for the Sarcoidosis. Before her scheduled hip surgery she was back in the hospital with other medical issues. Therefore she could not have the surgery. She then took more medications, which lead to more medications, and suffered, in extreme pain. All these illnesses had left her incapable of her daily activities, while she experienced excruciating pain throughout her body.

Mother had a fear of convalescent homes and did not want to go there as a patient. She had ministered to the people there on Sundays and did not like what she saw. We tried not to put her in one but were faced with the same problem we had with dad. As she became bed ridden and needed twenty-four hour care, we hired home care help and worked evenly with them. But it was a chore getting her to doctors' visits and caring for her so we were forced to put her in a convalescent home. On her second day there I went to visit her and was shocked at what I saw. She lay naked in the bed, mom who was so private and never wanted anyone to see her naked. My heart broke. I tried to be calm as I called the nurse to get her dressed. Later I reported it to the supervisor, who apologized and said it would not happen again.

Throughout her stay in the convalescent home my heart broke many times. Watching different aides clean her after a bowel movement knowing how she hated it, her being of sound mind and a strong mouth yet unable to help herself, and listening to her complaints about the pain. Sometimes I walked in to find her lying alone crying. We visited often bringing her flowers and fruits; her favorite was grapes. We also spoke to her on the phone everyday but she would still ask us, "When am I going home?"

Thanksgiving was the hardest because she had made it our family reunion. She took pleasure in setting the table with her best china, decorating it with candles and floral arrangements some of which she made herself. The gathering of all her children with their spouses and her grand children in her home gave her the optimum happiness. She was a good cook and her homemade eggnog was the best tasting eggnog one could find anywhere. Since we could not get her home for Thanksgiving we asked for a room at the nursing home and brought in the food. They had the perfect room, large with a fridge, microwave, a counter, two long tables and enough chairs for our big family. She thought it would not work but it was just like having it at home. She sat in her wheelchair and had a great time then thanked us.

Her stay in the convalescent home was short, about one year and four months. On December 3, 2002 she had her second cataract surgery. On December 4th, I went with her to the doctor for post surgery check up. An aide from the convalescent home was with us so I told her I would leave her with the aide and go run some errands while she waited for her ride back to the home. She said, "You are not going anywhere." Realizing that she was lonely I stayed. We sat and talked for a while as we waited for the van to arrive. We talked about the deficit in Connecticut and she asked that I bring her big coat for her next doctor's appointment. Finally her ride arrived and I said goodbye. That was our last talk and I felt happy that I had stayed with her that day.

The following day, December 5, 2002 I got a call from my sister AlvaJoy early in the morning saying that mom was found unresponsive in her room at the convalescent home and had been rushed to the hospital. One of her brothers had arrived that same morning from

Jamaica to visit her. He never got to have a conversation with her. The doctor said she had an infection in her eye, blood and urine. She was put on life support to help her breathe due to respiratory failure. None of the antibiotics they gave her could cure the infection. Once again my heart broke from seeing her with the tubes in her mouth, unable to talk, and swollen because she was retaining water.

It wasn't until December 10th, that she made her first contact with us by opening her eyes and nodding her head. Every day we went to the Intensive Care Unit with the hope that she would be better yet got only bad news that she was worse. The doctor had a meeting with us on December 20, 2002 to inform us that she would not leave the hospital alive and recommended we remove the life support machine. This was a tough decision for us to make. We discussed it, some agreed, some did not. Seven days later we decided that her suffering should come to an end. We had the hospital shut the machine off on Friday December 27th and on Saturday December 28, 2002 at about 8:55 p.m. she died. My sister Shirley had asked me to sit by mom's bedside with her, but I did not want to see mom die so I said no. My brother Hugh sat with her. At that time I was sitting at my desk at home doing some paperwork. I suddenly stopped, looked up in the left corner of the ceiling and thought about mama. The phone immediately rang and Shirley on the other end said, "Fay, Mama just died." I believe her spirit had visited me.

The following morning Sunday December 29, my brother-in-law in New York called to inform us that his wife, who had been as ill as my mother for some time, had died at 7:00 a.m. We now had two funerals back to back in the family. When my brother Harold spoke at mama's funeral his speech opened my eyes to how powerful she was. She was a mother, a father, dressmaker, business woman, and teacher simultaneously.

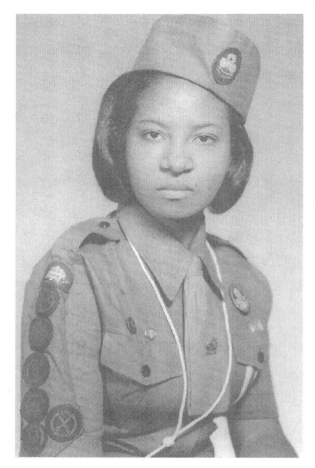

Figure 24: Fay as Girl Guide

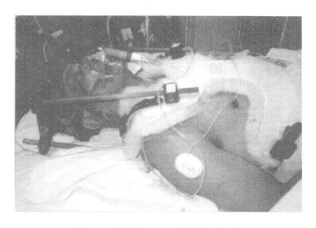

Figure 25: Papa with the halo

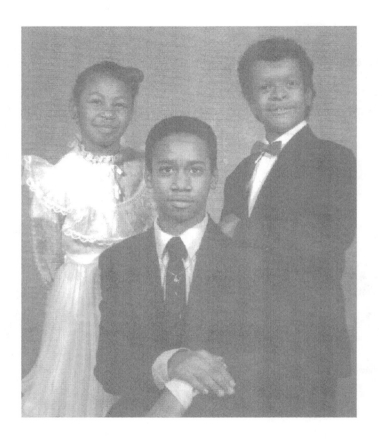

Figure 26: Monique, Charles Jr., and Sean.

CHAPTER 11

MY CHILDREN

I knew from a young age that I wanted four children, two boys and two girls. What I didn't know was that being a mother would cause such tremendous change in me. Motherhood transformed me from a naïve, quiet person into a strong, smart, mature woman.

My first child was hyperactive; I knew from my pregnancy that he was different. I asked other mothers if that was how their babies constantly moved in their bellies, they said yes, but after other pregnancies I discovered that was not true. Sure the other kids moved, but not as much. When Charles Jr. was born he was the only child in the nursery constantly kicking and moving. I would tell family and friends who came to visit that they should look in the nursery for the baby who was kicking.

Our first day home from the hospital was almost tragic. I kept him wrapped in the blanket because that is how all the babies were wrapped in the nursery. This would have been the right thing to do if it was winter or if there was air conditioning in the apartment. However, it was one of the hottest days in July, probably eighty degrees. The baby would not cease crying. His little brown face turned as red as an apple while his body became as hot as fire. The three people I called for advice all said the same thing, "Maybe he is hot, take off all of his clothes." The first person was an older woman with four children she also said to call the doctor. I told her he was too young to be naked he might get sick. The second person was my sister Georgia and finally the pediatrician. I removed the blanket. Georgia came over straight from work, stripped him, took his temperature, which was very high, gave him a bath and left him in his diapers only. Someone said he drew the hot temperature from the room as babies usually do.

The days that followed were like being in school. I learned new things on caring for my baby daily, mostly from my mother. The best moments for me and the baby were the ones we spent together late at nights to early mornings while his dad slept and I sat breastfeeding him, holding his little hand in mine looking down at his face as he suckled himself to sleep. The worst moments were the ones when his diaper was dry and his stomach was full yet he refused to stop crying. At times like these I would walk the floors with him, bouncing him and patting his back.

He grew up just as active, running around the apartment and wherever he went. His father liked playing music and as soon as the music started to play he started dancing crazily from one end of the room to the other.

I never forgot the time that I took him to the pediatrician and he kept sliding out of my lap and pulling the magazines off the table onto the floor. A woman sitting in the waiting room observing could not restrain herself from making a remark. She said, "He sure keeps you busy doesn't he?"

When it was time for him to be potty trained he would put the potty on his head and defecate on the floor. He must have been about three years old when I gave him a tricycle to ride outside around the apartment. I stepped inside for a minute and he disappeared. While I was searching and yelling for him, a woman brought him to me saying she had found him riding on the busy main street, about four blocks from where we lived. He said he was riding to McDonalds.

Shopping in the supermarket with him was impossible because when I put him to sit at the top section of the shopping cart he would stand. So I put him into the bottom with the groceries; then he threw the groceries on the floor. Finally, I put him on the floor to walk with me and he wants to run. Once, I let go of his hand to take an item off the shelf and he disappeared. As I searched the store from the meat section to the detergents and back again I saw a woman bringing him in from outside saying she found him in the parking lot.

When his brother Sean was born he loved the baby. As Sean grew up they played well together. One warm day in May, all three of us were in the kitchen; Sean was about three years old and Charles would be five that July. I was using the *Crazy Glue®* when my mother-in-law who was visiting called me into the living room. I placed the tube of *Crazy Glue®* on the table and walked into the room. As I entered the living room I heard Sean scream from the kitchen. I ran back into the kitchen and saw Sean with his hands covering one of his eyes as he bawled hysterically. "What happened?" I yelled. Charles Jr. said he thought it was eye drops so he dropped some into Sean's eye. His eye instantly glued shut. I rushed to the emergency room with him. The doctor said he could not open it. He recommended an ophthalmologist in another town. I dashed there immediately but he said he could not open it either. For over one week I searched for an ophthalmologist who could open my son's eye with no success. One problem was that they were afraid of damaging his pupil. Someone told me to put a washcloth with warm milk on his eye, but that caused infection. He started walking around the house like a blind child, holding onto the walls for guidance.

Finally, someone told me about an ophthalmologist at the Children's Hospital who might be able to open his eye. The day that I went there they were having a fair outside on the hospital grounds and most of the staff and patients were outside enjoying the food, music and games. The doctor was in his shorts having fun but he immediately escorted us to his office, where he opened my son's eye. He then dropped some eye drops into his eye and gave me some to take home to continue using for a while. He did not ask me about any health insurance until he was finished. This was the first and last time I had been to a doctor who did not inquire about health insurance before attending to the patient. That stuck in my mind. All the other doctors I had been to wanted insurance information first. Sometimes even before getting to their office their secretary wants all insurance information on the phone at the time of making the appointment.

A few years later, on a rainy day, Charley was babysitting the boys and he took them to my mother's house because he was helping her to paint a room. As the rain poured outside and Charley painted inside, I have no idea what my mother was doing; Charles Jr. took his brother, Sean with him and they went for a walk in the rain. Charley told me the story when I got home. He said he called the police and reported them missing. The police then told him that a woman had reported finding two boys walking alone and he should go to her house to identify them. When Charley arrived at the woman's house he saw them sitting on her bed dressed in her children's clothes. She had changed their clothes because they were wet from walking in the rain. If she had decided to keep them we would never have found them because she was Hispanic and they looked like Hispanic kids.

The first school Charles Jr. attended was a Catholic school. While he was there he would either get demerits or I would receive phone calls from his teachers about his activity almost every day. The school psychologist eventually informed me that the teacher had put him to sit in the hallway during classes; therefore her advice was to send him to another school. Finally, I took him to the children's hospital to be checked. The doctor diagnosed him with Attention Deficit Disorder (ADD) and suggested I put him on Ritalin. After asking about the side effects of the Ritalin, I declined when the doctor told me that the child could lose his appetite, suffer form insomnia or have a tic. He then suggested the school put him into a smaller, structured class. I removed him from that school, bought the "Feingold Cookbook for Hyperactive Children" and changed his diet by eliminating artificial colors, preservatives and sugars. For example, Kool-Aid, sodas and sweet cereal were no longer on his menu. The child calmed down. He had graduated from high school and trade school where he learned to fix computers along with other machines and was working in a job that he loved when I heard on the radio that Ritalin was the cause of death of some children. It was at that time I also learned that many children were taking drugs for behavioral problems.

In April 1977 my second son was born. Every

mother assumes that their baby will be healthy. Imagine my shock when the doctor broke the news to me that my baby was born sick and had to remain in the hospital for a few days. The pain of having to leave my newborn baby and go home alone was unbearable and I cried for many hours starting from the hospital. Not believing that pediatrician's diagnosis, I contacted another pediatrician for a second opinion. I was more devastated when he confirmed what the first one had said. During his stay in the hospital, I went there to breast feed him several times per day and decided to stay home for one year to care for him, working only on Saturdays since Charley would be home on the weekends.

According to the doctor the seizures the baby had was caused from his head being squeezed in the birth canal. He said he should take the Phenobarbital prescribed for the seizures for the rest of his life. However, a miracle happened when my mother anointed his little body with olive oil and prayed for him. On his next visit to the pediatrician, the pediatrician said the baby could stop taking the Phenobarbital. Added to this miracle, the child grew healthy and defeated most of the medical problems that faced him.

He was not as active as his older brother and was more obedient. The first time I told him to bring me diapers, he brought it right away and I was shocked because his brother did not listen to me. When I told Charles Jr. to do something I had to say it at least twice before he did it.

In 1980, our beautiful daughter, Monique entered into this world. When the nurse told me that I had a beautiful girl, my thoughts were, I don't think so, her nose is too flat. Then as she grew older I saw her turn into one of the most beautiful girls in the world. Sean told me that he was upset about the new baby because he had been getting all of the love before she came home and she was now taking the attention away from him. She was a well behaved child, so different from Charles Jr. She was quiet, loving and obedient.

She was about three years old when I put her in the bath tub half filled with water to give her a bath. I went into the bedroom to get her pajamas from the chest of drawers and got carried away fixing the clothes in the drawer being the neat freak that I am. When I went back into the bathroom she was under the water drowning. I was so frightened that with the speed of lightening, I nervously grabbed her out of the water shaking her, screaming her name, hugging her wet body close to mine, shaking and screaming again and again until I saw her gasping for air. What a relief that was when she started breathing normal again. I never left kids alone anymore, and do not like baby-sitting for other people because children are swift and you have to keep your eyes on them constantly.

The first time I dropped Monique off at a baby sitter we were both crying. My heart was broken having to leave her crying because she did not want to stay with the strange woman, but as duty called and I had to go to work I had no choice.

Being a mother with three children, I transferred to the night shift working from 7 p.m. to 7 a.m. three days one week and four days the next week. My plan was to care for the children in the days but I had forgotten about sleeping after work. The boys went to school all day but my daughter went for only half a day so I had to stay awake to pick her up at noon. After picking her up, I prepared lunch for her, brought it into the bedroom, locked the door, turned on the television, instructed her to watch it and eat whenever she got hungry then I went to sleep. I did not get enough sleep because she often interrupted my sleep by opening my eyes as she asked, "Mommy are you sleeping?" Some days I fell asleep while waiting for the time to pick her up and slept past the time. When this happened the teacher would call, very upset saying that Monique was the only child left in the school. Sometimes she threatened to take her downtown to the board of Education for me to pick her up there. The ridiculous thing was that she had to pass by my house to take the child to the board of Education but she could not stop to drop off the child at the house. Many nights I dragged myself to work very tired from lack of sleep, but I survived.

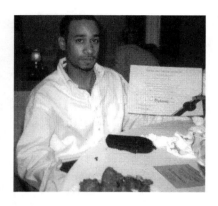

Figure 27: Charles Jr.

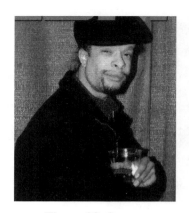

Figure 28: Sean

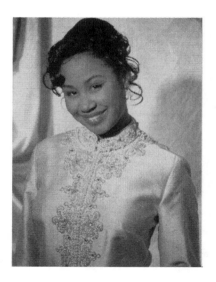

Figure 29: Monique

CHAPTER 12

THE APPRECIATION DINNER

I n the midst of my busy schedule, financial burden and physical pain, I took some time to fulfill a promise I had made to myself when I was lying on my back in Gaylord Hospital. Due to the overwhelming support I had got during my calamity, I concluded that the best way to show my appreciation to my family and friends would be to have an appreciation dinner and award them with certificates. Who would ever have thought that giving such a dinner would be a chore? The same people who dropped everything and helped me when I was sick could not find the time to come and accept my gratitude.

The list had soared to over one hundred people. Setting a date to fit everyone's schedule became a problem. Some were available for a said weekend but others were not. Finally August 8, 1992 was the date that everyone agreed on. Since I wasn't able to cook, I hired a caterer, the cost was per person. For this reason I requested an RSVP on the invitations. Many people responded. However, as time passed, new appointments filled in where my dinner invitation had been, yet only a few people informed me. My brother-in-law and his wife were the first two to tell me they would be in London on that date and would not be attending. One friend said an appreciation dinner was not necessary; a thank you was enough so she was not going to attend. One other friend told me she would be out of town. Arrangements were made for the others who were sure that they would attend.

My plan to keep it in the yard was perfect. Friends, family and acquaintances were excited. My sister AlvaJoy did the landscaping, decorating with new pots filled with the most beautiful *Impatiens* and *Geranium*. She placed white rocks and cider mulch around the roses, the flowers by the mail box, the flowers that lined the walkway leading to the house, the flowers surrounding the bird bath and around the flower beds that dotted the green grass on the lawn.

Among the flower beds I was going to put chairs and round tables for eating. The long tables I would set up in the garage to accommodate the food. The caterer would place a decorated arch and two pedestals at a designated area on the lawn. Under this beautiful arch there would be a table with a guest book where guests would sign their names before being seated. I had considered renting a tent, but declined after investigating the cost, it was too expensive.

Chairs and tables were already rented, wine and liquor were already purchased, and everything was finalized for Saturday August 8, 1992, when my husband Charley read the Old Farmer's Almanac and told me that it predicted rain for that weekend. Weekend includes Saturday and Sunday, but for some stupid reason I concluded that it would rain on the Saturday and not the Sunday so I changed the date to Sunday August 9, 1992. This meant renting a hall and calling everyone to tell them of the change. At this point I discovered some were not coming. One man said that he had surgery on his eyes and they were hurting, another was repairing his dentures and could not come without them. One woman was going out of town to a retreat and another was already out of town visiting her sick mother.

On Friday the 7th, I made arrangements to rent the West Indian Social Club to have the dinner there. With friends who were members of the Club, this was accomplished easily on such short notice. The second thing to do was to cancel the chairs and tables that were rented. The disappointment continued when the man in charge of renting me the club said I could not bring the liquor that was already bought, but had to use their bar at an extra cost. Along with this news he informed me that one of my very good friends would be leaving on a bus trip to Washington D.C., and would not be at the dinner.

Saturday August 8, 1992, turned out to be one of the most magnificent days God had ever created. It was a cool summer day with golden sunshine, the flowers smiling and the birds singing. This was a perfect day for anything. My heart almost failed from the anger I felt within for changing the date. I tried to console myself and waited to see what the following day would be like.

Sunday August 9, 1992 was born with a storm. It started while we slept and was expected to continue all day. The starting time was four o'clock; usually people are late, now everyone streamed in at exactly four p.m.; everyone except the caterer. I became nervous and asked around if anyone knew the reason why he was not there as yet, but no one knew. In the mean time three friends from work arrived. They were not dressed semi formal as I had requested on the invitation (they said it wasn't on theirs) so they became embarrassed because everyone else was dressed semi formal and they decided to leave. I spent some time trying to persuade them to stay since they were already there, but they insisted on leaving, so they left. It didn't matter to me how they were dressed; I only wanted their presence therefore I was very disappointed when they walked out the door.

Finally the caterer arrived. Later my husband told me that the caterer had encountered some problems on his way to the club. Before the food could be served one couple told me they had to leave because of another engagement at their church. I had planned to surprise them with a certificate of appreciation; I had to give it to them before the time. This put a damper on the surprise and my feelings were hurt.

When the dinner finally got started it went smoothly. Mother blessed the food and thanked God that we were all gathered there. My son Charles played the music. My daughter Monique played two songs on her saxophone, my brother-in-law Norris sang the lovely hymn "I will walk with God." Charley gave a toast and I gave my speech and handed out the certificates. Some people responded with a short speech about how long they had known me and that they liked my good attitude and friendliness. My nephew Gregory videotaped the complete dinner.

The family had advised me not to bring my father to the dinner since his sickness was unpredictable. Although I felt guilty and really wanted him there, I took their advice. Remembering how he had passed out at my brother Hugh's wedding the previous year causing a commotion when he fell to the floor (everyone probably thought he had died), I realized that they were right. He stayed home with the homemaker.

CHAPTER 13

JOURNAL

The year 1993 was one of the roughest years because I was still having bad pains in my back and my father needed lots of attention along with my mother and children. During this period I kept a journal. The journal will explain the hell I went through with my father, my family and my health.

January 25, 1993 Monday

It's a new year with the same old problems. Today I must get a paper signed for Papa, pick up his pills, bank his money and pick up Monique at Girl Scout meeting.

February 3, 1993 Wednesday

Pick up and cash papa's check, pay his rent, fill his pillboxes. Take Sean to Karate at 6:00 p.m. Monique to modeling meeting at 7:00 p.m.

Taylor

March 3, 1993 Wednesday

Another busy day: See Dr. M at 11:00 a.m. to get a filling in my tooth, pick up papa, cash his check, buy his pills, bring him home, take Sean to karate 5:30 p.m. and Monique to modeling meeting.

March 10, 1993 Wednesday

My mother's back is hurting badly. I must take her to see Dr. K, keep my appointment with Poquonock School for Monique's conference and take Sean to karate.

March 24, 1993 Wednesday

Mom's back continue to hurt so I must take her to see a chiropractor in Simsbury today.

April 7, 1993 Wednesday

My back was hurting extremely bad making it hard for me to walk.

April 12, 1993 Monday

Today is a very sad day for many people, young and old. It's the funeral of one of my children's schoolmate who was stabbed to death by another schoolmate. My children and I attended the funeral.

May 1, 1993 Saturday

Another sad day for me, it's the funeral of a friend of mine who died after a long illness. It's one of the biggest funerals I have ever attended. Police led the procession and there were cars for miles ending with another police escort. It is also the first funeral that I have been to where the burial was in a mausoleum instead of a grave.

It was during this funeral procession on May 1, 1993 that my second car accident occurred (the first car accident happened before the horse accident about 1988 as I was leaving work one morning. A woman reversed into the rear door of my car in the garage then told her insurance company that I had run into her). All the cars had stopped, the driver behind me did not notice because as he said, he was busy picking up a tape that fell. Since my car was not damaged, I did not call the police. Approximately two days later I had a stiff neck filled with pain, diagnosis was whiplash. This whiplash put me back into therapy for about one year.

The owner of the other car had no insurance therefore my insurance paid my doctor bills and I ended with a very small settlement again.

June 29, 1993 Tuesday

The numbness in my left leg started yesterday. Today it's worse; I am extremely frightened because the numbness has taken control and there is no sensation. Sitting on my bed observing the atrophy that started about two weeks ago, with no feelings and weakness I worry that soon I won't be able to lift it.

Saturday August 21, 1993

A woman pushed my father down in his apartment.

Thursday, August 26th

I took him to the doctor, then to take x-rays. They showed that his 9th rib was broken.

Friday, August 27th

Papa was worse than yesterday. I had stopped by his apartment with my son Sean on my way from the hospital where I had taken him for his regular visit. I brought papa home with me because I did not want to leave him alone sick in his apartment. Papa's medical doctor arranged for a visiting nurse, who met me as I was leaving with him. He was so weak he could not go upstairs for the interview. We all sat in the car by the side of the road while she tested and questioned him. He had a temperature. The visiting nurse will start on Monday along with the Meals on Wheels but he must stay at my home for the weekend.

Saturday August 28, 1993

After taking the Tylenol with codeine that the doctor had prescribed, Papa became very sleepy and unresponsive. I called my sisters Georgia (at work) and Shirley (at home) for help. Shirley came over.

Sunday August 29, 1993

At 4:00 A.M. I awoke to go to the bathroom; I went downstairs to check on Papa, he was o.k. I woke him about 10:00 A.M. to

165

brush his teeth. After staring around the bathroom for about five minutes, he asked for his toothbrush that was in his hand. It took about twenty minutes for him to complete this regular activity. He didn't eat much of his breakfast, only half of the cup of coffee and the glass of orange juice. He did not want to take a shower; instead he went back to bed. Two hours later he sat up and asked for his shower, which my son Sean helped him to do.

Monday August 30, 1993

I brought Papa to his home today but he could not make it upstairs so he waited for a half an hour before going up to his apartment. He was still weak and sleepy when the nurse took his blood pressure, and his temperature. Once again he was on his way to my home with me.

Tuesday August 31, 1993

I have three appointments today. See Dr. G. at 10:10 a.m. for my neck, an attorney at 12:30 p.m. and at 1:30 p.m. with Andrew from the local community homemaker program to discuss getting Papa home help or into a convalescent home, we decided on home help.

Wednesday September 1, 1993

My intention was to keep Papa home with me, but when the homemaker from the local community homemaker program called at 10:00 a.m. and said the home help and the nurse would meet him today at 1:30 p.m., I hurriedly brought him to his apartment to meet with them. I left him at 3:00 p.m. and at 5:00 p.m. his friend Bob called to tell me that he fell down and was on his way to the hospital in an ambulance. On my way from the modeling meeting with my daughter I stopped at the hospital and saw him in the emergency room. Nothing was wrong with him but I brought him home with me again.

Thursday September 2, 1993

Take Sean to the doctor at 9:30 a.m. then to the dentist at 12:00p.m. Georgia will take Papa to the doctor at 11:30 a.m.

Friday September 3, 1993

The home health care will start today for Papa.

Taylor

Monday September 13, 1993

Another rough day, after running from the post office, to the bank, to the modeling school, and the court I returned home to a message on my machine from Kathy the manager of the building where papa lives. It said, "Fay you need to come over here and see your father, he has been falling all day. He needs to be with you or in the hospital." I called my sisters Shirley and Georgia. Shirley met me at his apartment. We gave him dinner, cleaned up the place and left him looking good in his bed. The homemaker will be there in the morning.

Thursday September 16, 1993

Only three days later, Bob, his best friend in the building called. He said papa does not feel good and wants to see a doctor. When Georgia went to get him, she found him lying on his back. The kettle on the stove was still whistling.

Sunday September 19, 1993

My daughter and I stopped by to visit dad after visiting my mother who is not to be forgotten, she now has the shingles and need help. As we walked in my daughter exclaimed, "What's wrong with your face Papa?" He had three cuts on his face. I guess he was shaving himself. I went to make him coffee and found water in the bottle of coffee. He said he made a mistake by putting the water in it.

Then he had me searching all over for one foot of his socks, which was already on his foot, because he had both socks on one foot.

Monday September 20, 1993

The local community homemaker program awakened me. The homemaker could not get in, could I meet her there at 11:00 a.m. to let her in the apartment. Luckily I got him on the phone which saved me a trip to his apartment.

Throughout the month of September 1993, there were many calls from the local community homemaker program saying I should open the apartment for the homemaker to get in. On September 22, 1993, one of those early calls came while I was on the other line with the orthodontist making an appointment for my son whose braces had broken for the second time in four days. I angrily told the woman I could not meet her there because I had my own business to take care of. However, I calmed down and let her in before rushing to the orthodontist with my son.

When we entered the apartment we noticed the burn spots on my father's face as he said, "Let me show you what happened." We were shocked at what we saw. The oven door was completely off; his glasses under it and him saying that he can't find them. The oven was black inside and out, pots and pans were scattered over the kitchen counter. I went on to my appointment with my son while Georgia tried getting him out of the apartment but not without a fight. He thought he was going to the nursing home. LaVerne kept him at her house that night. The following day, September 23, Georgia spoke with the doctor, who suggested she take him to the emergency room so he could be thoroughly checked. On her way to the hospital with him he passed out three times. One was at the front of the hospital. Once inside he complained of dizziness and chest pains, and said he had hit his head the previous day. We felt some relief when he was admitted.

I was out of the house by 8:30 a.m. on Friday

September 24 to open the door for the homemaker so that she could clean up the mess. I then proceeded to therapy for the whiplash I had sustained in May. I returned to the apartment to see the homemaker off and continued to the hospital to visit papa. My arrival was at 12:00 p.m. and he asked me, "Why did you come so late?" Saturday September 25, the family learned of the blood clot in his head and his heart blockage. We left the hospital at 7:00 p.m., by 11:00 p.m. Georgia called to say that he had fallen in the bathroom at the hospital and hit his head; he got three stitches.

I could not visit on Sunday September 26, 1993 due to the excruciating pain in my back, the miserable feelings and the damp rainy weather. When my sister Babylin and I visited on Wednesday September 29, he did not recognize us.

Monday October 4, 1993 was another memorable day; mom called from the doctor's office, she was very sick and was admitted to the hospital. I got there in time to ride the elevator with her to her room. Both my parents were in the same hospital at the same time. After mom had settled in my sister LaVerne and I visited papa. He still did not recognize us. He was confused, spoke nonsense, chewed on the straw like a child and scraped the table with the fork when he tried to feed himself. LaVerne fed him and as we left the room he continued talking, nothing but nonsense.

Wednesday October 6, 1993 found them still in the hospital, dad still confused because of the blood clot in his head and mom not breathing properly. Georgia and I filled out an application at Kings Convalescent Home for dad.

Friday October 8, 1993, shocked at mom's condition this day. A change for the worse, along with the poor breathing she now feels weak. I went to therapy for my neck and shoulder before visiting both my parents. Being very tired on October 9, I decided not to visit, but when I heard that two of my sisters were working and a third was sick, I asked my daughter Monique to accompany me for the visit.

October 11, 1993 was the date dad went from the Ford Hospital to Kings Convalescent Home. He was immediately restrained because he continued to fall whenever he stood up. No one knew why he kept falling and he could not understand why he was being tied down. Mom went home from the hospital the next day and I was exhausted from all the errands. Georgia and I packed dad's belongings at his apartment and gave notice to vacate the premises on December 1st, with only one day to clear everything out.

December 24, 1993 dad and mom had dinner at my house then opened their gifts. Later I brought him back to the convalescent home. December 25, 1993 Dad had dinner at Shirley's house with the family while my family and I went to my uncle in New York for Christmas dinner. December 26, 1993 my brother Hugh had dad at his home for dinner. My father died seven years after his accident. And the water from the broken pipe continued to flow in my life getting dirtier as the years changed their numbers. Each year new problems arose, and they came in groups.

CHAPTER 14

MORE CHALLENGES

S ickness and accidents have become a way of life for me. When someone calls with the news, I am not shocked or surprised, you see, I get these calls almost every day. My family and I live the unexpected daily.

Charley and I were awakened early one morning with a call from his brother in Jamaica. A car had killed his five-year-old son. This brother had six boys. The youngest was taken early and a few years later another call came, another son had died at the age of seventeen. Thanks to cancer that has claimed so many lives. It was their faith in God that kept the parents of those boys moving on with their lives.

The first call we received from Jamaica in February 1992, said that my uncle was very ill and in the hospital. In March 1992, we received another call saying my grandmother had fallen and broken her ankle. The first week in April my uncle's wife called from New York and said that my uncle was admitted into the hospital. The second week of April my sister Georgia was admitted into a local hospital in Hartford. Five days later my sister AlvaJoy who lived in Waterbury called and said her father-in-law had died. About May 18th another call came from Jamaica, my grandmother was very sick in the hospital and knew she was dying. She wanted to see all her children and grandchildren before she died, could we come at once.

We had planned to leave on June 10th, but another call came on May 25th. My aunt said, "Come now, immediately, or you will see the body leaving the hospital in a bag." We booked an emergency flight and a group of twelve left for Jamaica on May 29th. I had heard of people waiting to see their family before they die but this was my first experience. Our return flight was on Friday June 5th 1992 at 5:00 p.m. Driving from New York I reached my home in Connecticut at 4:00 a.m. on Saturday June 6$^{th.}$. Sunday June 7th 1992 at 7:00 a.m. the call came from Jamaica, my grandmother, Agatha G, my mother's mom had died about 5:30 that morning. Although we had made funeral arrangements before we left Jamaica, my mother returned for the funeral. The following year, 1993 my only aunt who had called us with the information about my grandmother, fell sick suddenly and died. My mother went back to Jamaica for another funeral.

At one point I felt crushed. My life had been like a ship upon the rough sea being tossed to and fro, sometimes losing its direction but still moving. The constant changing of events gave me a choice to curl up and die or to move forward. I choose to use optimism as a weapon to fight my arduous life.

After the car accident in May 1993, my left shoulder continued to hurt. During October of "93" I was in and out of therapy when a plantar wart developed on the bottom of my right foot. Although I had surgery to remove this wart it continued to hurt and kept growing scar tissue. Each time the doctor removed the scar tissue it got sore and the pain increased making it hard for me to walk. This went on for several months.

On June 11, 1994 I received a call that had me rushing to my mother's house. Mom lived on the second floor and she was in the house and heard a crash, then felt it shake like there was an earthquake. She ran downstairs and saw a jeep lodged into her front porch. The fence, shrubs and front porch lay flat on the ground. I heard that it was a stolen jeep that was driven by an uninsured teenager. Since he had no insurance she had to pay for all the damages.

June 12, 1994, the night before my appointments with the orthopedist about my left shoulder and with the podiatrist about the plantar wart on my right foot, my left foot slipped off the chair pin and connected with the island kitchen table. I knew then that my big toe was broken because of the extent of the pain at the time of impact. Unlike others seeing stars, I saw a black cloud. The following day the orthopedist diagnosed bursitis in the left shoulder and a broken big toe on my left foot.

On retiring to bed at nights I had to massage the left shoulder with liniment, wrap the broken toe as directed by the doctor, dress the plantar wart, take the Advil for the pain and lie on the heating pad to soothe the lower back pain. This was after taking the Seldane for my allergy.

While waiting at a stop light on September 1, 1994, a wheelchair van reversed, smashing into the front of my car wrecking the vehicle. A few hours after being home my entire back began to hurt. I immediately called my medical doctor. He told me to sit in a tub of hot water, take some Advil and watch it. The next morning while still in pain I called him again and he said the same thing. I went to the emergency room after several failed attempts to see another doctor. The diagnosis was back strain; I was put on bed rest with medication and told to lie on the heating pad for fifteen to twenty minutes four times daily. During this time I had lost my sensation to void and my legs had gotten weaker.

My husband was celebrating his 50th birthday with a big party on September 4. I was on bed rest and could not help with entertaining or cooking. I felt useless as I lay outside on the lounge chair watching everyone having fun.

Later I went to my medical doctor who gave me prescriptions for pain and muscle relaxer then sent me to take x-rays. The doctor who read the x-rays advised me to go and see my orthopedist because a couple of the screws holding the rod in my back were broken. My orthopedist put me back in therapy, saying that he would not rush me into surgery.

The year 1995 opened with a line of illnesses steadily flowing through the year. My mother was about to go into the hospital for surgery when we heard that one of my nephews was in the hospital in Jamaica. Immediately after my mother returned home from having her surgery, my uncle in New York who had visited her in the hospital was now himself admitted. At the same time two of my sisters were home with bronchitis. About a week after my uncle returned home another nephew went into the hospital with pneumonia.

Then on November 10 1995, while at a McDonalds drive through window waiting for a sandwich, I was rear-ended sustaining whiplash again. The woman who hit me said her foot had slipped off the brake. This accident aggravated my neck and shoulder injuries, and put me into therapy for years. The woman's insurance refused to pay so four years later they had a jury trial. The morning of October 1, 1999, I was in court at 9:30 a.m. for the second pretrial for the case of the wheelchair van.

I was in the process of having the two cases within the same time frame. One case was scheduled for pre-trial in the morning with the hope of settling without a trial. Unfortunately, the other case that I refer to as the 'McDonald's Case' was scheduled for jury selection afterward. Sitting on the stand, I was made to feel like a criminal by the defendant's lawyer. Their doctor testified that I could not have been hurt from such a mild hit and while they were convincing the jury that I was not hurt from that accident my shoulder was killing me with pain. I lost the case and walked out of the courthouse in physical and mental pain, disappointed and empty handed.

The owners of the wheelchair van had accepted liability, but said my pain and suffering wasn't worth much, since I had been badly hurt before in the horse accident. Their insurance company dragged the case for five years, before sending me to their doctor for an independent medical evaluation. Although they were ten days late in sending me for this evaluation, the judge said I should still go. Their doctor, I will call him Dr. Kim, sent me a letter requesting that I bring in all my X-rays at the time of the visit. When I went to pick up the X-rays, the person in the department informed me that Dr. Kim already had the 1993 ones for the past three months.

At the evaluation I asked to see the X-rays, when he showed it to me he said, "Your screws were broken from 1993." Once again shock took control and I said nothing, because the first time I was told about the broken screws was in 1994 after the wheelchair van accident. I started investigating. The woman in the X-ray department said it should have been written in the report that accompanied the X-rays. After getting a copy of the report, I discovered that it was not written in the report. I contacted the doctor who read the X-rays in 1993; he casually said he must have forgotten to put it in the report that the screws were broken. Not only did he forget to write it in the report, he also forgot to mention it to me.

After Dr. Kim said that the screws were not broken because of the accident with the wheelchair van, they offered a small settlement. My attorney advised me to take the amount they offered. Everyone I told about the two cases said they never heard of two cases running at the same time for the same person with the same lawyer. My attorney said the judge would not allow her to change the date on the second case. It is my opinion that I will not die from an accident; neither will I be rich from the result of one.

Looking back at 1996, it was a great year. Although extremely busy, there were many good times. Between doctor's visits, therapy sessions, school meetings for my daughter, meetings at the convalescence home for my father, attending school and fundraisers, there were some fun times. The summer included four cookouts, some parties, a concert and a play. The play "Miss Saigon" was one of the best I had seen. Charley and I took a short vacation in Florida where we visited many friends and family members although they lived miles apart. It was on that trip that I worked on and completed the article "Life After Spinal Cord Injury," which was published in *Woman* magazine in Connecticut.

Later I took a trip to Virginia to visit my son Charles who had moved there, and then a cruise to the Islands with my two sisters Shirley and LaVerne. While on the cruise I missed many interesting events due to my dysfunctional bladder. It seems like half the time was spent in the bathroom. This was the year I turned fifty and my family threw me a big surprise birthday party. The weather was bad that night, it rained heavily with lots of flooding, but many of my family and friends braved the weather to celebrate with me. Some had arrived from New York the previous night and stayed at my mother's house to avoid being caught in the flood. It turned out to be a great party. The year 1996 was a fantastic one. Thank God for the experience and God bless my family for their help, support and love.

Just when I thought the road was smooth another pothole appeared. In April of 2001 I went for therapy as I usually do when the pain gets unbearable, only this time I had to go to another rehabilitation center because my new insurance did not participate with the center that I had been going to before. The therapist used the ultrasound machine on my back and after three treatments my left foot became as stiff as board and felt as if there was a tight band tied around it. I told the therapist that the ultrasound machine was not for me because my foot felt numb after he used it he said that the ultrasound was not the cause so he used it again. My foot got worse making it impossible for me to walk and I started falling around the house. In one of my falls I broke my little toe.

I could no longer walk with my straight cane and had to get a walker. I stopped the therapy and started seeking help from other doctors. My chiropractor who had treated my neck was surprised that the therapist had used that machine on my back. He said he should not have used it because of the rod in my back. The ultrasound produces heat and we do not want the rod to get heated; it could damage the nerves. The orthopedist and neurosurgeon said this is not true. They sent me to take CAT scan, X-rays, Mylogram and an EMG, a nerve test in which they stick me with needles to find damaged nerves. All tests were negative and they did not find any new nerve damage but I continued to deteriorate. The stiffness moved up to my leg and thigh and also on my big toe of my right foot. The muscles in my thigh and leg were so tight it felt like a permanent muscle spasm. I needed a wheelchair again.

Someone told me to see a Physiatrist; he sent me to the rehabilitation center that I had been going to before, prescribed pool therapy, and a foot brace. The therapist at the rehabilitation center taught me to walk with and without the brace, and sold me a walker with wheels that made me independent once again. This pulled more money from my already tight budget to pay for this walker because my insurance did not cover it. I must admit that I was angry at this new problem since I had been walking with a straight cane after leaving Gaylord. However, I learned to live with this new problem while working on regaining my strength and ability to walk without that walker again.

February 14, 2003 was a typical day. I did my daily routine; exercised, showered, had breakfast then ran my errands, returning home by lunchtime. After lunch I started having terrible chest pains. I thought it was acid reflux but four days later still in excruciating pain I rushed to my medical doctor who sent me to the emergency room. The doctor there also thought it was acid reflux; he gave me Pepcid and Tylenol and sent me home. Two days later still in pain I went to the gastroenterologist since some friends said it could be gallstones.   He sent me back to the emergency room where I was admitted.   After running several tests they said there were some gallstones but they were not the cause of my pain.

The diagnosis was Pericarditis, which is inflammation around the heart.   The doctors said I had picked up a virus that caused it.   They made a small incision in my chest and drained the inflammation from around my heart. When I awoke from surgery I discovered a tube in my mouth and my hands tied to the bed to prevent me from pulling it out.   Later more tests showed water around my lungs. They inserted a needle in my back to withdraw the fluid. After spending a week in the hospital I was admitted two more times with the pain.   The echocardiogram showed that some inflammation was still around my heart causing the pain. The doctors put me on medications and heavy doses of steroid and said it could take a long time to heal.

When I was leaving the hospital, a nurse gave me my discharge papers along with medications and instructions on how to take them.   One was the steroid called Prednisone, which I should take for two weeks only then go to my cardiologist Dr. Peters. On that visit Dr. Peters said the Pericarditis was not completely gone, therefore I should stay on the Prednisone. As the pain continued he increased the milligrams of Prednisone from ten to twenty then to forty. On forty milligrams of this steroid I had most of the side effects of the drug and could not stop taking it. Whenever I tried to stop by cutting the dosage, as I had to wean off, I got sick and had to increase it.

The first side effect I experienced was constant hunger. My stomach felt like an empty hole that could not be filled. While eating one meal I would be thinking of the next meal. This caused me to gain weight. A friend who was also taking it told me that while she was having one meal she was wondering what the next one would be. I was shocked and told her that the same thing happened to me. My food had no flavor, no taste. My face began to blow up like a balloon; some friends said it was called "Moon Face." Then followed the color change, my skin became yellow and spots appeared on some areas of my body. My beautiful black shoulder length hair came out in handfuls until the scalp appeared and there was no longer a ponytail. My blood sugar went up, my vision blurred and

I had to postpone my gall bladder surgery since the surgeon said Prednisone makes the body hard to heal after surgery. I did some research and discovered a more healthy way to heal myself. A friend of mine suggested I use a holistic treatment. After contacting a specialist in natural herbs I felt better, was able to stop taking the Prednisone, lost the weight gained from it, and also got herbs that prevented the need for surgery to remove my gallbladder.

Once again during this bout with the Pericarditis my family was there with me. My sisters took care of me, stayed in the room with me until late at night. My son, Sean came from Philadelphia where he lived and slept in the hospital room with me, my daughter visited from New York where she lived as often as she could, and my son Charles brought me food.

I believe it's a miracle that I had the strength to keep on going in my condition and thank God that I am still strong enough to help myself. At some point we were all on the other side of the bed. The circle of sickness continued with my sister Georgia, who had used her nursing skills to help us. It was now her turn to experience what mom; dad and I had been through. We thought we would lose her when a regular surgery turned into a nightmare. An infection developed that rejected all antibiotics. As in my case she was healed by a miracle through many people's prayers, it was not her time to die.

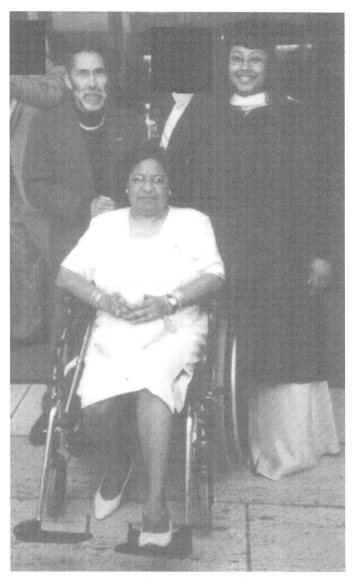

Figure 30: On Prednisone

189

CHAPTER 15

CONCLUSION

S ickness, accidents and death happen in every family. Not all at once, but eventually everyone will experience these. They are no respecter of person, place, race or age.   When they strike us we must try to handle the situation calmly, fix it to the best of our ability and continue on with our lives. We should not be stuck in one mode but should learn from the experience and make good from a bad circumstance. These things happen every day, we mostly hear about them on the news, sometimes it strikes a friend, or a neighbor, but what happens when they hit home? How do you deal with it? We never imagine that tragedy could strike us or our families and we are never prepared. Although they have been hitting my family and me for many years on a steady, regular basis, I am still not prepared to meet these unwelcome guests. What I have done is to deal with a situation as it occurs. Like a wall made of granite I am so strong that I can endure any bad news that is thrown upon me.

As a computer operator I worked with a Korean man who was given the problematic machines to work on regularly. He did not complain, he studied them and before long he knew everything about them and was able to fix them without calling the technician. Later everyone who encountered a breakdown with those same machines called on him. He always fixed them. He became a professional at operating and repairing them. I figure that if we approach life's problems in this manner we must conquer and survive.

I have certainly survived some of the toughest times in life, and in a way I am similar to the Korean man. He was called on to fix the broken machines. I am often called on to help others with their broken lives.

My hospital visits were so frequent it became a normal way of life. As soon as one person was out another was in. If I wasn't visiting, I would be waiting several hours in the emergency room. My family and I usually gathered in the patient's room bringing gifts, flowers and sometimes food. We talked, laughed, helped them and made parties from the visits. Our family's closeness helps us to cope.

Some of my time spent in the emergency room includes staying with my brother-in-law for hours until his wife arrived. Staying with my son who had a piece of glass fall into his eye from a broken ceiling light and on three different occasions staying all night with my daughter until morning when she was admitted, then continuing with daily visits until her return home.

On Thanksgiving Day 1998 my mother asked everyone present to say what he or she was thankful for. I liked what my brother Harold said best and will always remember his words. He said, "Thank God for all the challenges that this family has been given, because God knows we have had some big challenges." These words were another lesson for me. What we were having were challenges and we were handling them perfectly with God's help. No one committed suicide because it was too much to handle and no one started using cocaine to help them face the "problems." We kept on working, praying, helping each other and laughing through it all.

The course I had taken in reincarnation, explained that we have lived many lives because we must experience everything and one cannot experience everything in one lifetime. However, it seems that I am experiencing everything in this one lifetime. This includes sexual abuse as a child (I will not elaborate on this but I choose to mention it because it is a major crisis in my life that I have conquered), being raped as a teenager, not at the point of a weapon, but at the point of trust by men who I knew and trusted (one even drugged the drink he offered me), and mental pain as a young woman from married men posing as being single. I sometimes wonder why God allowed these things to happen.

I was exposed to many different religions at an early age. The church about a block from my grandmother's house was a small "Church of God Church," which drew my interest. I visited sometimes at nights, watching the people as they jumped and shouted, "Praise the Lord! Alleluia!" Some members of the congregation would hit their tambourines, others clapped their hands but they all sang and danced. Some got in the spirit and fell to the floor talking in tongues. The baptism was even more exciting. The covered pool under the floor of the church was opened. The people to be baptized were dressed in long, white gowns and the pastor held their clasped hands and the back of their necks then dipped them backwards in the water as he proclaimed, "I baptize you in the name of the father, the son and the Holy Ghost." I do not remember who took me there but someone had to have taken me because I was a child about eight years old.

Our yard was close to an intersection with two grocery shops. This corner was a meeting place for other religious groups. One could hardly get into one of the shops because of the crowd that was gathered on the piazza to listen to the Rastafarians. They praised Haile Selassie the former Emperor of Ethiopia saying, "Haile Selassie, King of Kings, Lord of Lords, Conquering Lion of the tribe of Judah, I and I Rastafari." The Rastafarians were easily recognized by their dread locks and long beards. This caused me to be afraid of them as a child. I enjoyed their meetings because they played drums and music that was pleasing to my ears and sang songs that were entertaining.

The other group that met at that corner was the Pukumina. They wore long white gowns and white pointed wraps on their heads, and jumped to the sound they made with their mouth.

I attended the Jehovah's Witnesses Hall with my aunt, the Baptist Church with my Grandaunt, and the Roman Catholic Church because my mother wanted me to go there. I did not understand some of the customs of that church, like why on entering the church did the people dip their hands into the water that was placed by the door and make the sign of the cross on their bodies? Why did they genuflect before entering their seats? Why were statues in the church? The Latin spoken by the priest sounded good but what was he saying? All this was a wonder for me as a teenager. I started to study the Catechism but left the church before it was time for confirmation and found my way to the Methodist Church. I liked their way of worship and was received into the church at seventeen years old. I loved attending church and hated to miss a Sunday. Feelings of guilt would ride my conscience all day if I missed a service. A voice kept saying, "You should have gone to church."

Although I loved going to church there were many questions in my mind about God. Who and where was God? How could people say they love God when they could not see God? Another thought was, how could God be in all of us and see what's happening everywhere? In school we prayed in the mornings before classes began. We prayed before leaving for lunch, also on returning from lunch and at the end of the day before dismissal. To this day the dismissal prayer is what I say at bedtime.

We had a class on Religious Knowledge that taught us Bible stories and the meaning of the parables that Jesus told. We also had to study passages from the Bible. We knew the twenty third Psalms by memory. I prayed for everything I wanted and had faith that my prayers would be answered because of what I had been taught, that God is our father who provides for us. I asked God if He was real to reveal Himself to me. This is one prayer I will always remember saying in church. All of my prayers were answered. It was no coincidence that certain books entered my life to help me understand the spiritual aspect of life. Revealing that God is a Spirit not a man sitting on a chair in heaven as I had imagined when I was a child.

Being optimistic and my faith in God have helped me to push the ugly things that happened aside and focus on the good ones. Sometimes I throw my little "pity party," feeling sorry for myself where the life I view as a bed of rose petals becomes the thorns on a rose bush. I have learned that life is like a bed of rose bushes with both the beauty of the petals and the pain of the thorns. We can choose to see only the flowers and remove the thorns when they hurt us or we can continue to hold on to the stems and be pricked by the thorns. We have a choice and since we will always have challenges we should let go of the thorns and move forward among the petals. As we walked through the rose garden at a park my sister Joy said to me, "I love roses, they remind me of life." I was astonished, because I thought that I was the only person who saw the comparison.

Many years have passed since my horseback riding accident. The permanent pain has made me a meteorologist predicting the weather better than the weather channel. This pain I have named the "Rain Pain." I have retired and turned to writing about my experiences. I consider it a blessing to be able to cope with the challenges in my life. I accept life for what it is: a mixture of good times with laughter and sad moments with tears. I feel that I have been tested with life's challenges and passed the test.

I survived it all and will survive any future challenges that will enter my life because I am strong mentally, physically, and spiritually.

APPENDIX

Cards and Well Wishes

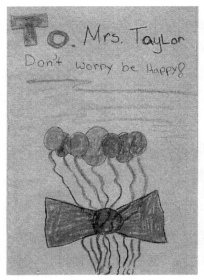

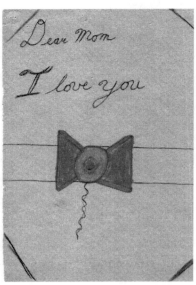

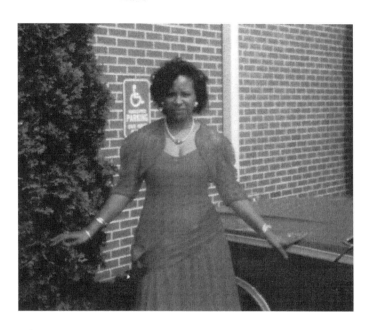

Ironically, Fay poses next to a handicap sign before the accident

Taylor

Excerpts from a company newsletter

Actuaries can tell you how many people will be injured in America each year through statistics. It is very unfortunate that they can't tell you who these will be as well.

Many of the people in Operations and APSU go out of their way just to say Hi to Fay Taylor. She is an Operator on shift 3 at the Home Office. Fay is one of the rare wonders still found in society today. A kind and gentle person. Her gentle smile and pleasant greeting help bring a little sunshine into any humdrum day. Fay has worked at […] for approximately 11 years and always has a kind word to say.

This past July, Fay became one of the statistics these actuaries calculate. She and her husband Charlie were on vacation in the Poconos when the horse she was riding spooked. Fay was thrown from the horse and her vacation was turned into a nightmare. Fay broke her back. During surgery, which lasted close to 12 hours, the doctors at Thomas Jefferson Hospital in Philadelphia restructured her back using a steel rod and a piece of bone taken from her hip.

Fay has since been moved to Gaylord Hospital in Wallingford. The long process of recovery and rehabilitation will begin there.

People such as Fay often go unrewarded for their virtues. We as Fay's friends and admirers do not want this to happen to Fay. A special fund has been set up to help Fay and her family with medical and rehabilitation costs. Those wishing to contribute please contact one of the persons listed below.

We miss Fay and wish her a complete and speedy recovery.

Fay's response printed in the company newsletter

Editors Note:
Below you will find a response from Fay Taylor on an article that was written on her in our last issue.

After reading that beautiful article about me in the last issue of [...] I would like to respond.

It really made me feel good that somebody thinks so highly of me. "One of the rare wonders of the world". (SMILE). I did not know that I was one. I always thought of myself as a foolish person because I smile too much, but that article made me think differently. However, I am a wonder to myself. My sister called me a 'saint'. My mother and husband said to me, "Fay cry or curse, do something! You are taking this accident too good." You see, after being to hell and back, I am still smiling. Lying here in a body cast from my neck to my knees, with my legs apart waiting for time to pass. The nurses and doctors cannot understand how I can take it so lightly and always greet them with a smile. I told the counselor I did not need him. He said "You may not need a counselor, but it's good to talk to someone." After a few weeks of talking to me he told me he told my husband I will heal fast because of my good attitude. To be honest, maybe I would not be smiling if the doctor had said I would be paralyzed. But when he said I will walk out of here, I had something to smile for. My family and friends were so supportive with their visits, cards, gifts, phone calls, flowers, and

Taylor

lots of love that I had something to smile for. I would like to take this opportunity to say thanks to *K and *D and to all my co-workers for their support, cards, gifts, and fruit baskets. That too was a reason for me to smile.

I am doing good, healing nicely and getting lots of therapy on my hands and legs. I am still in a cast but a shorter one which was put on in mid-October. After thinking about what could have been worse, I am still smiling because I have many reasons to smile. Thank God I am still alive and I am a strong person. I will be back!

FAY LINDO TAYLOR

About the Author

Fay Lindo Taylor was born in Kingston, the capital city of the idyllic island paradise Jamaica West Indies. Educated at Waulgrove College, migrated to the USA in 1970 in order to pursue upward mobility and broaden personal horizons.

After residing in Potomac, Maryland for a year and a half, living in New York for six months, relocated to Hartford Connecticut, where she met and married her devoted husband Charles A. Taylor. This special union produced and nurtured three amazing children-Charles Jr., Sean, and Monique.

Employed by Hartford Insurance Group in various computer technology positions until the tragic accident occurred in 1989. Now, retired and healing, has decided to share her life-altering experience to benefit and empower the quiet voices who have courageously endured and survived the devastation of Spinal Cord Injury.

The Learning Exchange, Editor Barbara Gershenbaum, coupled with English courses at Capital Community College and the Summer Program at Smith College were instrumental in honing and advancing her writing and academic skills.